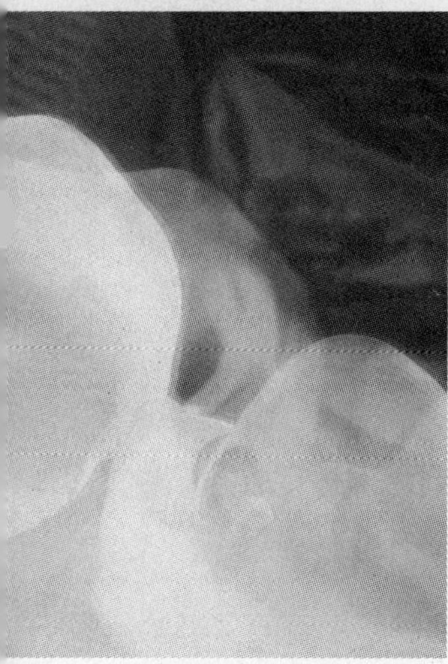

Study Guide

GLENCOE

Nursing Fundamentals

A Patient-Centered Approach

June Eastmond, BSN, MS, RN
Indian River Community College
Fort Pierce, Florida

Ethel E. Killgore Taylor, BSN, RN
San Antonio College
San Antonio, Texas

Elizabeth Yeh, BSN, MSW, RN
Western Career College
Sacramento, California

Consultants

Helen Greene, BSN, RN
Catawba Valley Community College
Hickory, North Carolina

Janet A. Lyons, BSN, RN
Director of Nursing, Split Rock Nursing Home
Bronx, New York

Glencoe McGraw-Hill

w York, New York
umbus, Ohio
sion Hills, California
ria, Illinois

ivision of *The* **McGraw-Hill** *Companies*

Glencoe/McGraw-Hill

A Division of The ***McGraw-Hill*** *Companies*

STUDY GUIDE
NURSING ASSISTANT FUNDAMENTALS: A Patient-Centered Approach

Send all inquiries to:

Glencoe/McGraw-Hill
936 Eastwind Drive
Westerville, OH 43081

ISBN 0-02-802425-7

1 2 3 4 5 6 7 8 9 POH 05 04 03 02 01 00 99 98 97

Co-developed by
Glencoe/McGraw-Hill
and Chestnut Hill Enterprises, Inc.
Woodbury, CT

Study Guide

GLENCOE

Nursing Assistant Fundamentals

A Patient-Centered Approach

CONTENTS

INTRODUCTION

The *Study Guide* for *Nursing Assistant Fundamentals—A Patient-Centered Approach* helps you review the information you have learned in the textbook and allows you to check off tasks as you perform them. This self-study process will prepare you for your certification examination as well as for your entry into the job market.

Each chapter of the *Study Guide* is divided into sections. Chapters without procedures have four sections, and chapters with procedures have five. The five sections are described below. When using the *Study Guide*, make sure you have read each chapter of the student text thoroughly before testing yourself. Finish each section before proceeding to the next.

Study Objectives

The study objectives give you a brief overview of the chapter and a few sentences about each objective in the textbook. The objectives outline the major points needed to master the content of the chapter. As you review each objective, evaluate whether you have mastered it. If you are not comfortable with your understanding, refer to the textbook, or check with your instructor for further clarification.

Know Your Terms

The second section of each chapter tests your knowledge of the key terms you learned in the textbook. Each key term is boldfaced in the chapter and also appears in the glossary that begins on page 663 of the textbook. Take the matching test without referring to your textbook. Check your answers in the answer key, which begins on page 277 of the *Study Guide*. If you have mastered all the terms, go on to the next section. If not, carefully review each term you missed until you feel you have learned it.

Matching exercises for chapters with many key terms have been divided into two or three parts to make studying more manageable. Do each matching exercise, check the answers, and review as necessary.

Test Your Knowledge

The next section, Test Your Knowledge, tests your understanding of the major concepts of the chapter. Each chapter has ten questions. Answer the questions with your textbook closed; check your answers in the answer key that begins on page 277 of the *Study Guide*, and, if you have missed any, reread that section of the textbook, or check with your instructor before proceeding.

Think About the Issues

As a nursing assistant, you will make many choices and you will think over many issues that will confront both you and the patients you serve. This section of the *Study Guide* asks you to focus on some issues you may face and to practice thinking through the critical personal and health care decisions that you and people in your care will face. For the most part, the answers to the questions in this section are personal and need not be shown to anyone. You may choose to discuss some of the issues with your fellow students, or you may wish to ask instructors for guidance in some cases.

Check Your Skills

The last section of each chapter of the *Study Guide* gives you a task checklist for each procedure in the textbook. Some procedures start with the following boxes:

Standard Precautions	☐ Handwashing	☐ Gloving	☐ Gowning	☐ Masking
Introductory Tasks	☐ Gather Equipment	☐ Identify/Introduce/Explain		☐ Provide Privacy

First, put a checkmark in each box that applies. You may have only one checkmark (for example, almost all procedures require handwashing), or you may check all seven boxes. Before you actually perform procedures, it is assumed that you will know how to implement standard precautions, gather equipment, communicate clearly with patients, and provide privacy where appropriate. These tasks are not individual to each procedure.

Some procedures do not contain a box section because the boxes do not apply. In these cases, go directly to the numbered tasks. When you check *yes* next to a task, you are affirming that you have performed that item to your own satisfaction and in accordance with the rules you have learned. When you check *no* to a task, make sure to review with your instructor how you can improve your performance.

Depending on the type of program in which you are enrolled, you may check the tasks with your instructor or by yourself. A comment section below each procedure leaves space for the instructor to write notes about the procedure to help you remember key steps. You may also use this section to write down personal reminders about the particular procedure.

In most states, you will be tested on some, if not all, of the procedures. Mastery of the tasks that make up each procedure is essential to your mastery of the job of nursing assistant.

CHAPTER 1

THE NURSING ASSISTANT

STUDY OBJECTIVES

The nursing assistant is a member of the health care team who is usually supervised by a licensed nurse. Caregivers in long-term care facilities need certain qualities to be successful. They also need to understand the regulations that govern their jobs and the scope of practice for their field.

- Nursing assistants need to be honest, dependable, conscientious, empathic, patient, helpful, professional, objective, and have a positive attitude in order to provide the highest level of care.
- Health care teams may consist of only two people—a caregiver and a client—or they may consist of many staff members in many different fields. The patient is always the most important member of the team.
- Nursing assistants provide personal care and aid in the activities of daily living for residents, patients, or clients. They also keep rooms safe and clean. They take and record vital signs. They provide nutrition and assist in therapy and rehabilitation programs.
- The scope of practice for nursing assistants includes limitations. They may not give or prescribe medication, diagnose illness, or perform sterile procedures. They are also bound by ethics and the limits of their job to respect patients' privacy and not to comment on diagnosis or treatment.
- OBRA regulations set the standards for the job of nursing assistant. They also list the specific skills that must be mastered before a nursing assistant can work in a long-term care facility.
- Nursing assistants maintain their own personal health and hygiene through proper diet, cleanliness, adequate sleep and rest, reasonable exercise, and the avoidance of unsafe behaviors.
- Home health aides provide care to clients who are ill, but who are able to live at home.
- Home health aides may do food shopping and preparation, laundry, and some cleaning.
- People interested in nursing assisting as a career should express an interest in giving care, particularly to the elderly population.

KNOW YOUR TERMS

In the space provided, write the letter of the definition that best fits the numbered term.

__ 1. caregiver	a. An act establishing the minimum federal requirements for nursing assistants.
__ 2. charge nurse	b. The allowed tasks for a specific job.
__ 3. conscientiousness	c. An ability to wait and to bear difficult situations and people.
__ 4. dependability	d. A person who is trained to give basic personal care in a health care facility.
__ 5. empathy	e. The attribute that means a person can be relied on.
__ 6. head nurse	f. Services in a region or in a health care facility that promote social well-being.
__ 7. health care team	g. Willingness to provide aid and support (as in a 1 caregiver situation).
__ 8. helpfulness	h. A work ethic that includes careful and honest attention to all aspects of a job.
__ 9. home health aide	i. A nurse who has completed a one- to two-year training program and has passed a state licensing exam.
__10. honesty	j. A trained health care provider who carries out the orders of doctors, gives medications, performs some treatments and therapies, and may set up care plans.
__11. licensed practical nurse (LPN)	k. Another term for nurse.
__12. licensed vocational nurse (LVN)	l. All those involved in making and carrying out health care decisions.
__13. nurse	m. Another name for charge nurse.
__14. nursing assistant	n. The ability to perceive something as it is without injecting personal feelings or prejudices.
__15. objectivity	o. One who provides care.
__16. Omnibus Budget Reconciliation Act (OBRA)	p. The quality of being fair and straightforward in dealings with others.
__17. patience	q. An attitude that shows optimism in dealing with others and a willingness to perform one's daily tasks without complaint.
__18. positive attitude	r. The conduct that meets the standards of a profession.
__19. professionalism	s. A nurse who has completed a nursing program taught either in public vocational high schools or other state-approved programs.

__20. registered nurse (RN)	t. A person who works as a caregiver in home health care.
__21. rehabilitation	u. A nurse who is head of a department and who supervises other nurses.
__22. scope of practice	v. The process of restoring someone to their prior or best capacity after an injury or illness.
__23. social services	w. The ability to understand and indirectly experience the feelings, thoughts, and difficulties of others.

TEST YOUR KNOWLEDGE

Write the word(s) that best completes the statement.

1. Two basic qualities needed by nursing assistants are _____________ and _____________.
2. A _____________ worker follows instructions carefully and thoroughly.
3. The most important member of the health care team is the _____________.
4. Providing basic care is usually the task of the _____________ _____________.
5. Nursing assistants are not allowed to administer _____________.
6. It is the responsibility of doctors to _____________ illness.
7. Federal requirements for nursing assistants are given in _____________.
8. Good personal hygiene helps control the spread of _____________.
9. A nursing assistant who wants to work part-time may work as a _____________ _____________.
10. The demand for nursing assistants is _____________.

THINK ABOUT THE ISSUES

1. Avoiding unsafe habits is important for your own health and for the health and safety of patients in your care. Review your personal health habits and list ways you can improve them.
2. What is your personal attitude toward work? How do you think your attitude will affect your job performance?

CHAPTER 2

WORKPLACES IN THE HEALTH CARE INDUSTRY

STUDY OBJECTIVES

Nursing assistants work in different types of health care workplaces. The patients, residents, or clients they care for also differ. Hospitals, subacute care units, and skilled nursing facilities care for people with a variety of illnesses. Recuperative facilities, such as convalescent homes or rehabilitation centers, work on restoring people to their best possible state of health. Cost factors in health care today are changing where, how long, and from whom people can receive health care.

- The major types of health care workplaces are hospitals, nursing homes, clinics, convalescent homes, and home health situations.
- Patients in hospitals and subacute care units are generally sicker and need more care than people in other facilities. People in assisted-living facilities or group homes usually take care of many of their own needs. Clients in home care are often independent. People in nursing homes often need help with most aspects of their daily care.
- Nursing assistants in long-term care facilities provide basic personal care and care of residents' rooms.
- Cost-cutting measures in health care include earlier release from hospitals, greater numbers of people in managed care, and the employment of fewer high-level professionals.

KNOW YOUR TERMS

In the space provided, write the letter of the definition that best fits the numbered term.

__ 1. adult day-care center	a. A residential facility that provides care for people with chronic disorders or disabilities or who are unable to care for themselves.
__ 2. assisted-living facility	b. A home that serves as a residence for several people with disabilities, mental retardation, or mental illness.
__ 3. client	c. A facility that provides medical or surgical care.
__ 4. clinic	d. A residential complex, usually for the elderly or people with disabilities, where residents live in their own units but where additional health care services are provided as necessary.
__ 5. convalescent home/ convalescent hospital	e. A center that attends to the needs of adult (usually elderly) clients during the day.
__ 6. group home	f. A unit in a long-term care facility that takes care of patients who are too ill to be in the general population but who have been released from the acute care of a hospital.
__ 7. health maintenance organization (HMO)	g. A person receiving health care services.
__ 8. hospice	h. Health care funding for people over 65 and for certain disabled persons.
__ 9. hospital	i. Another name for a long-term care facility.
__10. long-term care facility	j. A facility for the medical treatment of patients or clients.
__11. managed care	k. A health care facility providing extended care for patients needing recuperation.
__12. Medicaid	l. A person receiving service from a health care provider, usually in a clinic or at home.
__13. Medicare	m. A person who lives in a place (in health care, a person who lives in a nursing home).
__14. nursing home	n. A facility or program that provides care for the terminally ill who have chosen to avoid extreme medical interventions.
__15. patient	o. A long-term care residence for people who are unable to care for themselves.
__16. preferred provider organization (PPO)	p. An organization that provides full health care to a group of subscribers in a certain geographic area.
__17. rehabilitation center	q. A group health plan where listed providers charge members of the plan lower than normal rates.

__18. resident — r. A health care facility specializing in rehabilitation.

__19. skilled nursing facility — s. Health care funding for the poor.

__20. subacute care unit — t. A group health plan that provides care from a pool of providers and facilities.

TEST YOUR KNOWLEDGE

Write the word(s) that best completes the statement.

1. Patients who are released from hospitals but who still need recovery care may enter the _____________ care unit of a nursing home.
2. A long-term care facility is also called a _____________ home or a _____________ nursing facility.
3. Care for people who live at home but need daytime supervision may be found in an _____________ _____________-_____________ _____________.
4. Hospice services are for patients who are _____________ _____________.
5. After a car accident, an injured person usually receives medical care in a _____________.
6. In home care situations, nursing assistants may do light _____________.
7. A group of doctors who sign agreements to work for a lower fee for a group of patients form a _____________ _____________ _____________.
8. Most managed care is provided in _____________ _____________ _____________.
9. Medicare provides health care funding for people over _____________.
10. Medicaid provides health care funding for the _____________.

THINK ABOUT THE ISSUES

1. Some managed care plans limit the types of treatments available. This means that some people may be refused certain treatments, but it also means that many more people get basic care. Do you think this is fair? Why or why not?
2. Working in hospitals can be interesting because of the variety of patients you see. However, most stays are short-term and you rarely get to form the same kind of relationship as you do in long-term care. Which do you think might work out best for you?

CHAPTER 3

LEGAL RIGHTS, ETHICS, AND COMMUNICATION

STUDY OBJECTIVES

People who receive care have all the rights and privileges of everyone else. Nursing assistants must respect those rights and should do every task in an ethical manner. They should also learn good communication skills for communicating with patients and fellow health care workers.

- Patients and residents have a right to good quality, respectful care, a right to freedom from abuse, coercion, or restraint, a right to privacy, a right to choose their own care, and a right to dignified treatment.
- Nursing assistants have the legal obligation to give care in a professional manner, to respect the people they give care to, and to always act in an ethical manner.
- Nonverbal communication includes facial expression, body language, appearance, and touch.
- Caring communication includes active listening, asking open-ended questions, and courteous speech.
- Some obstacles to good communication are asking "why" questions, using pat answers, and giving opinions or advice.
- Good phone communication includes speaking clearly and repeating any messages for confirmation. Answering an intercom also requires clear speaking. A call signal should be answered immediately or within a few minutes.

KNOW YOUR TERMS

MATCHING EXERCISE I

In the space provided, write the letter of the definition that best fits the numbered term.

__ 1. abuse	a. Questions that can be answered with only a yes or no.
__ 2. active listening	b. The process of giving and getting information.
__ 3. assault	c. A set of rules for proper personal and professional standards of conduct.
__ 4. battery	d. The willful mistreatment of someone (can be physical, mental, emotional, or sexual).
__ 5. choice	e. The body of law concerned with crimes.
__ 6. civil laws	f. The power to select.
__ 7. closed-ended questions	g. A communication skill in which the listener pays close attention to the speaker and shows keen interest by use of body language.
__ 8. coercion	h. An unsatisfactory condition or situation about which a formal complaint is made.
__ 9. communication	i. An attempt to force someone to do something against his or her will.
__10. confidential	j. The body of law covering individual rights and relationships among members of society.
__11. criminal laws	k. Secret; containing private information.
__12. defamation	l. Hitting or touching without a person's consent.
__13. ethical standards	m. A violent or threatening physical or verbal attack.
__14. grievance	n. Harming people's reputations by writing or saying untrue things about them.

MATCHING EXERCISE II

In the space provided, write the letter of the definition that best fits the numbered term.

Term	Definition
__ 1. health care proxy	a. Questions that encourage people to talk by requiring more than a yes or no answer.
__ 2. incapacitated	b. A person whose role it is to investigate complaints and issue findings about those complaints.
__ 3. informed consent	c. A statement signed by a patient or his or her representative giving someone power to make health care decisions in case of the patient's inability to do so.
__ 4. invasion of privacy	d. Any treatment given by trained health care providers that causes harm due to failure to follow accepted standards of practice, or by performing procedures beyond their training or authority.
__ 5. legal rights	e. Harm caused when a trained health care provider fails to perform in a reasonable, careful manner, according to accepted standards.
__ 6. living will	f. A violation of civil law that occurs when a patient is not protected from unwanted visitors or from unwanted release of confidential information.
__ 7. malpractice	g. A statement developed by the federal government as part of OBRA, setting forth the rights of people who reside in long-term care facilities.
__ 8. negligence	h. A document signed by a patient or proxy attesting that he or she understands and gives approval to a surgical or other medical procedure.
__ 9. nonverbal communication	i. Unable to function fully.
__10. ombudsman	j. A set of guidelines for patients and health care providers produced by the American Hospital Association.
__11. open-ended questions	k. A written statement about how someone wishes to be treated in the event of serious or catastrophic illness.
__12. Patient's Bill of Rights	l. Communication that takes place without speaking (as communication using body language, facial expression, and so on).
__13. Residents' Bill of Rights	m. The body of rights that the law provides to individuals.

TEST YOUR KNOWLEDGE

Write the word(s) that best completes the statement.

1. The freedom from being intruded upon is called the right to _____________.
2. An _____________ serves as a resident advocate.
3. Following the law is a _____________ concern for nursing assistants.
4. Following the standards of a profession is an _____________ concern for nursing assistants.
5. A gentle touch is one form of _____________ communication.
6. One form of caring communication is _____________ listening.
7. A _____________-_____________ question requires only a yes or no answer.
8. An _____________-_____________ question cannot be answered by a simple yes or no.
9. A _____________ _____________ _____________ may be assigned by patients to make medical decisions for them in case they become incapacitated.
10. Patients who are bedridden may summon help by using a _____________ _____________.

THINK ABOUT THE ISSUES

1. Why is it important to act according to the ethical standards of a profession?
2. Evaluate your own telephone communication skills. Do people seem to understand your telephone speech? Are they always asking you to repeat things?

CHAPTER 4

THE PATIENT

STUDY OBJECTIVES

Patients are people who have basic needs and special needs relating to their health problems and to the places where they are receiving care. Patients' cultural backgrounds should be understood and respected. Visitors provide important outside contact for patients.

- All people have basic needs including food, water, air, shelter, and clothing. Higher-level needs include security needs, social needs, esteem needs, and self-actualization needs.
- Nursing assistants generally help patients whose illness prevents them from taking care of their own activities of daily living. Nursing assistants often work with people who are elderly, who have a long-term disability, or whose mental condition prevents them from caring for themselves.
- Residents in long-term care facilities need encouragement to maintain a social life, to be as independent as possible, and to stay as active as possible.
- Home health care clients generally need help to stay at home. Nursing assistants may help with personal care, housekeeping, providing companionship, and feeding.
- Short-term care patients are generally ill or injured for a short time and need help in performing personal care tasks while recovering from their illness or injury.
- Patients' backgrounds may differ in their cultural beliefs, their practices, and their behavior.
- Patients' visitors need information about the facility, privacy with their family members, and a sense that the patients are receiving the best possible care.

KNOW YOUR TERMS

In the space provided, write the letter of the definition that best fits the numbered term.

__ 1. activities of daily living (ADL)	a. A state of feeling psychologically content and happy.
__ 2. acute	b. Of old age or aging.
__ 3. chronic	c. Basic human needs for food, water, air, sleep, elimination, and shelter.
__ 4. culture	d. Disease.
__ 5. emotional well-being	e. The general condition of the body; good general condition of the body.
__ 6. esteem needs	f. Physical tasks (mobility, self-care, grooming, dressing, and so on) necessary to maintain oneself.
__ 7. geriatric	g. The accumulation of customs, values, and objects shared by a people.
__ 8. health	h. Those needs that must be met in order to have a feeling of self-worth.
__ 9. illness	i. Following birth.
__10. obstetrical	j. Of or relating to the care and treatment of children.
__11. pediatric	k. The preparatory time before surgery.
__12. physical needs	l. Lasting a long time (said of an illness or condition).
__13. postoperative	m. A feeling of being able to form and maintain relationships with friends and family and to interact comfortably in social situations.
__14. postpartum	n. Of the medical practice that deals with pregnancy and childbirth.
__15. preoperative	o. The group of needs that, when fulfilled, allows a person to feel safe. These needs include security, stability, order, protection, and freedom from fear and anxiety.
__16. security needs	p. The group of needs that, when satisfied, makes a person feel accepted and loved.
__17. self-actualization needs	q. Having a life expectancy of less than 6 months.
__18. social needs	r. Brief, severe (said of an illness; not chronic).
__19. social well-being	s. Following surgery.
__20. terminal	t. These psychological needs that, when fulfilled, enable someone to reach his or her highest potential.

TEST YOUR KNOWLEDGE

Write the word(s) that best completes the statement.

1. All people need ______________, ______________, ______________, sleep, elimination, and shelter.
2. ______________ needs satisfy people's need to feel that they belong and are loved.
3. A disease that is always present is called a ______________ condition.
4. A disease of short duration is called an ______________ illness.
5. ______________ patients are over the age of 65.
6. A common mental disorder of people in long-term care is ______________ disease.
7. A person who is cared for at home may feel more ______________ than a person cared for in a facility.
8. The period after childbirth is called the ______________ period.
9. The accumulation of customs, values, and objects shared by a people is called their ______________.
10. Patients' ______________ usually provide support and care.

THINK ABOUT THE ISSUES

1. Other than meeting physical and security needs, which needs do you think are the most important, and why?
2. Name two things about cultures other than your own that make you uncomfortable. Name two things about your own culture that you think might bother other people.

CHAPTER 5

HUMAN GROWTH AND DEVELOPMENT

STUDY OBJECTIVES

As people develop, they go through various stages. During these stages, certain physical and psychological changes take place. Not every person experiences every stage at the same time or even in the same order, but the general path of human development is similar for most people.

- The stages of childhood include neonate and infancy, toddler period, preschool period, primary period, and preadolescence. During these stages the child grows and develops from a small, dependent being to a child who can take care of many of his or her own physical needs (bathing, feeding, walking, elimination, and so on). The child learns to communicate using language and develops emotionally.
- During adolescence, individuals usually grow to their adult size, shape, and sexual maturity. The conflict between the need for family support and for independence often causes family difficulties.
- During young adulthood, people usually establish their careers and families. Often, they leave their own families and set up their own homes.
- Middle-aged adults move from the peak of their careers to retirement. If they have children, the time of separation usually occurs during middle adulthood.
- The changes experienced in late adulthood are the physical changes of aging, which leaves some people debilitated and in need of care. Emotionally, late adulthood is a time to prepare for one's own death and the death of one's peers.
- Personalities mature as we age. If psychological needs are met consistently throughout life, individuals are able to reach a stage of wisdom in their old age.

▲ KNOW YOUR TERMS

In the space provided, write the letter of the definition that best fits the numbered term.

__ 1. adolescence	a. The process of going through the natural physical and emotional stages leading to maturity.
__ 2. development	b. The period of life after age 65.
__ 3. developmental tasks	c. The period of life from age 41 to 65.
__ 4. growth	d. The period of life from age 3 to 5.
__ 5. immunization	e. A set of tasks that must be accomplished to complete a stage of development.
__ 6. late adulthood	f. The period of life from age 6 to 9.
__ 7. menarche	g. The period of human development from age 13 to 18.
__ 8. menopause	h. The period of life from age 10 to 12.
__ 9. middle adulthood	i. An involuntary reaction in response to a stimulus.
__10. neonate	j. The accumulation of individual characteristics that distinguish someone or something.
__11. personality	k. The person who is mainly responsible for meeting a child's basic needs; the main caregiver for a person who is ill or disabled.
__12. preadolescent period	l. The period of life from age 1 to 3.
__13. preschool period	m. The ending of menstruation, usually in middle adulthood.
__14. primary caregiver	n. The stage during which a child develops secondary sex characteristics and becomes capable of reproducing sexually.
__15. primary period	o. The process of making someone resistant to disease (as by inoculation).
__16. puberty	p. The first menstrual period.
__17. reflex	q. The period of life from birth to 4 weeks.
__18. toddler	r. The period of life from age 19 to 40.
__19. young adulthood	s. The process of growth.

▲ TEST YOUR KNOWLEDGE

Write the word(s) that best completes the statement.

1. A baby who is between birth and 4 weeks old is a ______________.
2. The preschool period is from ______________ to ______________ years old.
3. Formal schooling begins during the ______________ ______________.

4. The stage in which the sex organs mature is called ______________.
5. The demand that group members of about the same age act alike is called ______________ ______________.
6. ______________ is a period that occurs during the teenage years.
7. During ______________ ______________, people establish themselves in their own work and family lives.
8. Women experience ______________ during middle adulthood.
9. Chronic conditions may be increasingly debilitating during ______________ ______________.
10. The sum of our behaviors and emotional characteristics is called our ______________.

▲ THINK ABOUT THE ISSUES

1. What do you remember as the hardest period of your life so far? Do you think old age will be easier?
2. Do you think adults can change their personalities?

CHAPTER 6

SAFETY

STUDY OBJECTIVES

Safety includes keeping patients safe, preventing accidents, acting properly in emergencies, and keeping yourself healthy and safe.

- To prepare for emergencies, learn all emergency procedures in a facility. In a home care situation, learn where emergency equipment is kept. Also, know where a telephone is located in case you need to call 911.
- Know how to evacuate patients in a fire emergency, how to extinguish small fires, and how to prevent fires from occurring.
- Knowledge of how to follow instructions in other emergencies and in health emergencies is essential to a health care worker.
- Weather emergencies require preparedness and an ability to follow instructions.
- A doctor might prescribe restraints for a patient in danger of falling out of bed or a chair, for a patient who cannot control aggressive action and is in danger of hurting him- or herself or others, or for a patient who may remove needed IV lines.
- Oxygen is flammable, so avoiding sparks or fires is essential to safe use of oxygen.
- Keeping personally safe on the job includes avoiding infection, using correct body mechanics to avoid injury, knowing fire safety rules, and watching out for potential safety hazards, such as a wet floor.
- Ambulatory patients should use hand rails, walking aids, and transfer belts when necessary. They should wear nonskid shoes or slippers, and their pathways should be kept clear.
- Standard precautions include handwashing, gowning, gloving, and masking, as necessary.

KNOW YOUR TERMS

In the space provided, write the letter of the definition that best fits the numbered term.

__ 1. ABC Class fire extinguisher	a. Able to walk or walk about; not confined to bed.
__ 2. aerosol therapy	b. A type of fire extinguisher used to control grease fires.
__ 3. All Class fire extinguisher	c. Therapy that delivers moisture or medication into the lungs in conjunction with oxygen therapy.
__ 4. ambulatory	d. An oxygen delivery device consisting of a plastic tube inserted into the patient's nose and connected at the other end to an oxygen source.
__ 5. Class B fire extinguisher	e. A fire extinguisher that can be used for any type of fire.
__ 6. Class C fire extinguisher	f. Another name for ABC Class fire extinguisher.
__ 7. croupette	g. An oxygen delivery device consisting of a two-pronged plastic tube inserted into the patient's nostrils and connected at the other end to an oxygen source.
__ 8. emergency	h. The four critical steps in a fire emergency.
__ 9. face mask	i. Railings attached to the side of a bed that can be raised to prevent falling out of bed.
__10. hand rail	j. An oxygen delivery device consisting of a face mask worn by the patient and connected to an oxygen delivery unit.
__11. heatstroke	k. A gaseous element necessary to sustain life.
__12. nasal cannula	l. Guidelines set up by the CDC for the prevention of infection.
__13. nasal catheter	m. A device that restricts movement, usually used only when safety concerns are involved.
__14. oxygen	n. Any sudden crisis calling for immediate action.
__15. P.A.S.S.	o. A type of fire extinguisher used to control electrical fires.
__16. R.A.C.E.	p. The sequence of critical steps when using a fire extinguisher.
__17. restraint	q. A small portable unit similar to an oxygen tent.
__18. side rails	r. A severe and possibly fatal condition caused by exposure to extreme heat and characterized by confusion and high fever, sometimes leading to coma.
__19. Standard Precautions (SP)	s. A set of CDC infection control guidelines, now replaced by standard precautions.
__20. Universal Precautions (UP)	t. A safety rail, usually in a hallway, for ambulatory residents.

TEST YOUR KNOWLEDGE

Write the word(s) that best completes the statement.

1. A potentially dangerous event calling for immediate action is an ______________.
2. The first thing to do in a fire emergency is to ______________ ______________.
3. The body's failure to regulate its internal temperature is called ______________.
4. A ______________ is used to keep patients from harming themselves.
5. The air we breathe is made up of 21% ______________.
6. The newest CDC guidelines are called ______________ ______________.
7. The most important procedure for preventing the spread of microorganisms is ______________.
8. Always wash your hands before putting on ______________.
9. Use a ______________ and a ______________ if blood or body fluids are likely to splatter.
10. Ambulatory patients should wear ______________ shoes or slippers.

THINK ABOUT THE ISSUES

1. A patient in restraints may be confused and angry. What can you do to make the patient as comfortable as possible?
2. If you think a patient does not have an infectious disease, should you use standard precautions anyway?

CHECK YOUR SKILLS

In the following procedure checklists, check each task box that applies and answer yes or no to each step you have completed. If possible, have your instructor sign off when you have completed a procedure.

PROCEDURE

USING A FIRE EXTINGUISHER

	Yes	No
1. Hold the fire extinguisher upright.	___	___
2. Remove the safety pin.	___	___
3. Direct the hose at the base of the fire.	___	___
4. Push or squeeze the top handle down to close.	___	___

Procedure Completed ______________________ **Date** ______________________

Notes ____

____

____

PROCEDURE

USING A FIRE BLANKET

	Yes	No
1. Roll the patient on his or her side, facing away from you.	___	___
2. Place the fire blanket diagonally under the patient. Roll the patient on his or her back.	___	___
3. Wrap the patient in the blanket. Wrap as you would wrap a blanket around a baby.	___	___
4. Lower the bed to the lowest position. Loosen the bottom bed sheet and use it as a sling to gently lower the patient to the floor.	___	___
5. Grasp the edge of the blanket. Get into a crawling position and pull the patient along the floor. Stay as low as possible when there is smoke.	___	___

Procedure Completed ______________________ **Date** ______________________

Notes ____

____

____

PROCEDURE

SP

APPLYING A WRIST OR ANKLE RESTRAINT

Standard Precautions ☐ Handwashing ☐ Gloving ☐ Gowning ☐ Masking

Introductory Tasks ☐ Gather Equipment ☐ Identify/Introduce/Explain ☐ Provide Privacy

	Yes	No
6. Position the bed to a comfortable working height.	___	___
7. Place the patient in a comfortable position with correct body alignment.	___	___

	Yes	No
8. Place the soft edge of the restraint against the patient. Place it over clothing or padding. Wrap the restraint around the wrist or ankle, and smooth the fabric of the restraint. Make sure there are no wrinkles.	___	___
9. Gently pull the ends of the straps through the fastening ring. Make sure the restraint is secure but not tight.	___	___
10. Test for proper fit by putting two of your fingers between the restraint and the patient. If your fingers do not fit, loosen the restraint.	___	___
11. Move the arm or leg into a comfortable position.	___	___
12. Tie the ends of the strap to the bed frame with a tie according to the facility's policies and procedures.	___	___
13. Check the pulse, color, and temperature of the patient's wrist or ankle.	___	___
14. Put the bed back to its normal position. Raise the side rails if ordered.	___	___
15. Give the patient the signal cord. Recheck the patient before leaving the room. Make sure the patient is comfortable.	___	___
16. Unscreen the patient.	___	___
17. Wash your hands.	___	___
18. Remove the restraint every 2 hours to reposition the patient. Provide patient care and exercise.	___	___

Procedure Completed ______________________ **Date** ______________

Notes ____

____

____

PROCEDURE

APPLYING A MITT RESTRAINT

Standard Precautions ☐ Handwashing ☐ Gloving ☐ Gowning ☐ Masking

Introductory Tasks ☐ Gather Equipment ☐ Identify/Introduce/Explain ☐ Provide Privacy

	Yes	No
6. Position the bed to a comfortable working height.	___	___
7. The patient's hands should be clean and dry.	___	___
8. Place a hand roll in the patient's hand so the hand is comfortable.	___	___

	Yes	No
9. Apply the mitt restraint. Tie the straps to the bed frame, according to the facility's policies and procedures.	___	___
10. Make sure the restraint is secure but not tight. Check the pulse, color, and temperature of the wrist.	___	___
11. Put the bed back to its normal position. Raise the side rails if ordered.	___	___
12. Check that the patient is comfortably positioned before leaving the room. Make sure the patient is positioned in correct body alignment.	___	___
13. Unscreen the patient.	___	___
14. Wash your hands.	___	___
15. Remove the restraint every 2 hours to reposition the patient and provide patient care and exercise.	___	___

Procedure Completed ______________________ **Date** ______________________

Notes ____

____

____

PROCEDURE

OBRA SP

APPLYING A JACKET RESTRAINT

Standard Precautions ☐ Handwashing ☐ Gloving ☐ Gowning ☐ Masking

Introductory Tasks ☐ Gather Equipment ☐ Identify/Introduce/Explain ☐ Provide Privacy

	Yes	No
6. Position the bed to a comfortable working height.	___	___
7. Assist the patient to a sitting position. Slip the armholes of the jacket on the patient's arms. Cross the straps over the patient's chest.	___	___
8. Help the patient to lie down.	___	___
9. Pull the loose end of the strap through the slot in the jacket, making sure there are no wrinkles in the jacket.	___	___
10. Place the patient in a comfortable position.	___	___
11. Tie the straps to the bed frame under the mattress.	___	___
12. Make sure the restraint is secure but not tight. Test for fit and comfort by inserting two fingers between the restraint and the patient. Put the bed back to its normal position. Raise the side rails if ordered.	___	___

	Yes	No
13. Give the patient the signal cord. Check the patient's position and comfort before leaving the room.	___	___
14. Unscreen the patient.	___	___
15. Wash your hands.	___	___
16. Remove the restraint every 2 hours to reposition the patient and provide patient care and exercise.	___	___

Procedure Completed ______________________ **Date** ______________________

Notes ____

____

____

PROCEDURE

APPLYING A SAFETY BELT RESTRAINT

Standard Precautions ☐ Handwashing ☐ Gloving ☐ Gowning ☐ Masking

Introductory Tasks ☐ Gather Equipment ☐ Identify/Introduce/Explain ☐ Provide Privacy

	Yes	No
6. Position the bed to a comfortable working height.	___	___
7. Assist the patient to a sitting position.	___	___
8. Place the safety belt across the front of the patient's waist. Pull the ties to the back.	___	___
9. Pull the ties through the slots in the belt. Smooth all the wrinkles from the fabric of the restraint.	___	___
10. Help the patient to lie down.	___	___
11. Place the patient in a comfortable position.	___	___
12. Tie the straps to the bed frame under the mattress.	___	___
13. Make sure the restraint is secure but not tight. Test for fit and comfort by inserting two fingers between the restraint and the patient. Put the bed back to its normal position. Raise the side rails if ordered.	___	___
14. Give the patient the signal cord. Check the patient's position and comfort before leaving the room.	___	___
15. Unscreen the patient.	___	___

	Yes	No
16. Wash your hands.	___	___
17. Remove the restraint every 2 hours to reposition the patient and provide patient care and exercise.	___	___

Procedure Completed ______________________ **Date** ______________________

Notes ____

____

____

PROCEDURE

APPLYING ELBOW RESTRAINTS

Standard Precautions ☐ Handwashing ☐ Gloving ☐ Gowning ☐ Masking

Introductory Tasks ☐ Gather Equipment ☐ Identify/Introduce/Explain ☐ Provide Privacy

	Yes	No
7. Place the patient in a comfortable position with correct body alignment.	___	___
8. Wrap the restraint around the patient's elbow. The restraint is placed on top of clothing, pajamas, or padding.	___	___
9. Tie the straps around the arm.	___	___
10. Secure the restraint to the patient's shirt with the safety pins or Velcro straps.	___	___
11. Repeat steps 8 through 10 to apply the restraint to the other elbow.	___	___
12. Check the restraints for proper fit. They must be secure but not tight.	___	___
13. Give the patient the signal cord.	___	___
14. Place the patient in a comfortable position.	___	___
15. Unscreen the patient.	___	___
16. Wash your hands.	___	___
17. Check the patient every 15 to 30 minutes.	___	___

Procedure Completed ______________________ **Date** ______________________

Notes ____

____

____

PROCEDURE

OBRA SP

STANDARD PRECAUTION: HANDWASHING

	Yes	No
1. Push your watch up your arm or remove it. Push your sleeves at least 4 inches above the wrist.	___	___
2. Using a dry paper towel, turn on the faucet. Make sure your hand does not come in direct contact with the faucet or sink. Adjust the water until it is warm. Dispose of the paper towel.	___	___
3. Wet your hands. Keep your fingertips pointed downward.	___	___
4. Take the soap from a dispenser. Use enough soap to create lots of lather.	___	___
5. With your hands pointed downward so water does not run up your arm, rub your hands together in a circular motion. The act of rubbing your skin together creates friction, which loosens microorganisms. Rub vigorously for 60 seconds (or for as long as your facility requires). Clean each wrist. Clean under your fingernails and around each nail.	___	___
6. Rinse your hands with warm running water. Continue to hold your hands down, allowing water to flow off the fingertips. Take care to remove all soap from your hands.	___	___
7. Dry your hands and wrists with a paper towel. Do not shake fingers or hands. Discard the paper towel without touching the waste container.	___	___
8. Turn off the faucet with a clean paper towel and discard the towel immediately. Make sure your uniform, hands, and wrists do not directly touch the faucet or sink.	___	___

Procedure Completed ____________________ **Date** ____________________

Notes ____

____

____

PROCEDURE

OBRA SP

STANDARD PRECAUTION: GLOVING

	Yes	No
1. Remove your jewelry.	___	___
2. Wash and dry your hands.	___	___

	Yes	No
3. Slip your hands into the gloves, one hand at a time. Be careful not to tear the gloves on your fingernails. If your facility requires that you use double-gloves, place a second pair of gloves over the first pair.	___	___
4. Do not wear torn gloves. Inspect your gloved hands before administering patient care.	___	___

Removing Gloves:

	Yes	No
1. The outside of the glove is contaminated. Do not touch any part of your own skin with a gloved hand.	___	___
2. Pinch the inside of one glove at least 1 inch below the cuff.	___	___
3. Pull the glove down and over your hand so that the glove is inside out.	___	___
4. Hold the glove completely inside the hand, which is still gloved.	___	___
5. Place two fingers of the ungloved hand under the cuff of the glove.	___	___
6. Pull the glove down and over the hand, so that the first glove is completely inside the second glove.	___	___
7. Dispose of the gloves in an appropriate waste container.	___	___
8. Wash your hands.	___	___

Procedure Completed ______________________ **Date** ______________

Notes ____

____

____

PROCEDURE

OBRA SP

STANDARD PRECAUTION: GOWNING

	Yes	No
1. Remove all jewelry and watches. Roll up your sleeves.	___	___
2. Wash and dry your hands.	___	___
3. Hold the clean gown in front of you so it unfolds. Do not shake the gown.	___	___
4. Slip your hands and arms through the gown, making sure the gown completely covers the front of your uniform.	___	___
5. Tie the neck strings.	___	___
6. Overlap the back of the gown and tie the waist strings in the back.	___	___
7. Make sure the back of your uniform is completely covered.	___	___

	Yes	No
Removing the gown:		
1. Remove your gloves (if still on) and wash your hands.	___	___
2. Untie the waist strings.	___	___
3. Wash your hands.	___	___
4. Untie the neck strings. Do not touch the outside of the gown.	___	___
5. Pull the gown off your shoulders by the ties. Reach under the cuff of each sleeve and pull the gown off each arm.	___	___
6. Roll the gown up away from you, turning it inside out.	___	___
7. If paper, dispose of the gown in a waste container. If cloth, put it in the appropriate container for washing.	___	___
8. Wash your hands. Use a dry paper towel to open the door. Dispose of the paper towel inside the door as you exit.	___	___

Procedure Completed ______________________ **Date** ______________________

Notes ____

____

____

PROCEDURE

OBRA SP

STANDARD PRECAUTION: MASKING

	Yes	No
1. Wash your hands.	___	___
2. Pick up the mask by the ear loops or upper ties. Do not touch the piece that will cover your face.	___	___
3. Place the mask over your nose and mouth, making sure that both your mouth and nose are covered. (Never walk around hallways with a dangling mask.)	___	___
4. Pull the loops or upper strings over your ears. Tie the strings in the back toward the top of your head.	___	___
5. Tie the bottom strings at the back of your neck. If you wear glasses, the mask should fit snugly over your nose and under the bottom of the glasses.	___	___
6. Mold the metal strip over the bridge of your nose.	___	___
7. Wash your hands.	___	___
Removing the mask:		
1. Wash your hands.	___	___

	Yes	No
2. Untie the lower strings first, then the upper strings.	___	___
3. Bring the strings together to the front of your face. Do not touch the inside of the mask.	___	___
4. Dispose of the mask in a waste container.	___	___
5. Wash your hands.	___	___

Procedure Completed ______________________ **Date** ______________________

Notes ____

____

____

CHAPTER 7

EMERGENCY CARE

STUDY OBJECTIVES

Emergencies require clear thinking and quick action. Knowledge of emergency procedures can save lives. Weather and fire emergencies require knowing where to go and who to notify. Patient health emergencies require specific skills depending on the type of emergency.

- ▲ Patients may encounter weather and fire emergencies, cardiac or respiratory arrest, shock, stroke, bleeding, seizures, burns, choking, and poisoning.
- ▲ CPR is the resuscitation of someone who is in cardiac and/or respiratory arrest. Only a trained person should perform CPR.
- ▲ To perform the Heimlich maneuver, stand behind the choking person, put your hands below his or her sternum, make a fist with one hand and clasp it with the other, and give five upward thrusts.
- ▲ To aid a person in shock, first administer CPR and stop bleeding, if necessary. Next, raise the feet higher than the head and keep the person warm. Get help.
- ▲ A person who seems to be having a stroke should receive CPR, if necessary. Turn the victim's head to the side, elevate the head, and cover and keep the victim warm and calm until help arrives.
- ▲ When a person is hemorrhaging, perform CPR, if necessary. Put pressure on and elevate the wound. Apply a tourniquet, if necessary.
- ▲ Protect seizure victims from injuring themselves and keep them calm until help arrives.
- ▲ Burn victims must first be removed from the fire. Then, perform CPR, if necessary. Follow the procedures for the different levels of burns until help arrives.
- ▲ Call the poison control center and follow directions for a victim of poisoning.

▲ KNOW YOUR TERMS

In the space provided, write the letter of the definition that best fits the numbered term.

__ 1. cardiac arrest	a. A chronic brain disorder usually characterized by seizures.
__ 2. cardiopulmonary resuscitation (CPR)	b. Any substance that is toxic to humans.
__ 3. choking	c. A procedure for dislodging an item that is causing a victim to choke.
__ 4. epilepsy	d. A partial seizure characterized by blank staring and muscle twitching.
__ 5. external bleeding	e. Care or treatment given at the scene of an injury or illness.
__ 6. first aid	f. The part of CPR during which a rescuer forces oxygen into the victim's lungs.
__ 7. generalized absence seizure	g. A state in which a foreign object blocks air from entering the lungs.
__ 8. grand mal seizure	h. Another name for generalized absence seizure.
__ 9. Heimlich maneuver	i. A stopping of the heart.
__10. hemorrhage	j. A sudden physical or mental disturbance (as one caused by an injury, or by learning some terrible and unexpected news).
__11. internal bleeding	k. Something that a patient tells you he or she feels physically.
__12. petit mal seizure	l. Extensive discharge of blood (through blood vessels).
__13. poison	m. Something about a patient that you can see, hear, or feel.
__14. rescue breathing	n. Another name for tonic-clonic seizure.
__15. respiratory arrest	o. A method of restoring breathing after a cardiac arrest by putting pressure on the chest and supplying mouth-to-mouth respirations at regular intervals.
__16. shock	p. A cerebrovascular accident.
__17. sign	q. The point at which breathing stops while the heart continues to work for a few minutes.
__18. stroke	r. A signal to show that one is choking, made by clutching the neck with one or both hands.
__19. symptom	s. To bleed on the outer surface of the body.
__20. tonic-clonic seizure	t. Bleeding inside the body, beneath the surface of the skin.
__21. universal distress signal	u. A strong seizure characterized by convulsions.

▲ TEST YOUR KNOWLEDGE

Write the word(s) that best completes the statement.

1. When breathing stops, the patient is in ____________ ____________.
2. ____________ ____________ occurs when the heart stops.
3. ____________ ____________ combines rescue breathing and external chest compressions.
4. The ____________ ____________ has saved many people from choking to death.
5. A patient in shock should have the feet put ____________ than the head.
6. A cerebrovascular accident is also called a ____________.
7. Apply ____________ to a wound that is spurting blood.
8. A ____________-____________ seizure is more serious than a ____________ ____________ seizure.
9. A ____________-degree burn is much more serious than a ____________-degree burn.
10. A ____________ is any substance that can change the function of body organs and adversely affect the patient's health.

▲ THINK ABOUT THE ISSUES

1. You may not always be able to use standard precautions in an emergency. If you cannot, should you help save someone in spite of the risk to yourself?
2. Some people ingest poisons in an attempt to commit suicide. Do you think that these people should be allowed to die? Should age be a factor?

▲ CHECK YOUR SKILLS

In the following procedure checklists, check each task box that applies and answer yes or no to each step you have completed. If possible, have your instructor sign off when you have completed a procedure.

PROCEDURE

OBRA

HELPING A CONSCIOUS PERSON WHO IS CHOKING

	Yes	No
1. Stand behind the victim.	___	___
2. Wrap your arms around the victim's waist.	___	___
3. Make a fist with one hand and place the thumb side just above the victim's navel and well below the tip of the sternum.	___	___
4. Grasp your fist with your other hand.	___	___
5. Press the fist into the victim's abdomen with a quick upward thrust.	___	___

	Yes	No
6. Give five thrusts. Each thrust should be a separate and distinct effort to dislodge the object.	___	___
7. After every five abdominal thrusts, check the victim and your technique.	___	___
8. Repeat cycles of five thrusts until: • the victim coughs up the object, or • the victim becomes unconscious , or • you are relieved by emergency medical personnel or another trained person.	___	___

Procedure Completed ______________________ **Date** ______________________

Notes ____

____

____

PROCEDURE

OBRA

HELPING AN UNCONSCIOUS PERSON WITH AN OBSTRUCTED AIRWAY

	Yes	No
1. Straddle the victim's thighs.	___	___
2. Place the heel of one hand against the middle of the victim's abdomen slightly above the navel and well below the sternum. Your fingers should be pointing toward the victim's head.	___	___
3. Place your other hand directly on top of the first hand.	___	___
4. Press inward and upward using both hands. Complete five quick abdominal thrusts. Each thrust is a distinct and real effort to relieve the airway obstruction.	___	___
5. After five thrusts, perform a finger sweep of the mouth. This is performed only on unconscious victims. Use your thumb and forefinger to grasp the victim's jaw and tongue and lift upward. This pulls the tongue away from the back of the mouth and away from a foreign object. **a.** With the index finger of the other hand, slide the finger down along the inside of one cheek. Go deeply into the mouth. Use a hooking action and move to the other cheek and up. **b.** If an object comes within reach, grab and remove it.	___	___
	___	___
6. If you are still unsuccessful, repeat the following cycle until you are relieved by emergency medical personnel or another trained person: • Give two rescue breaths • Perform up to five abdominal thrusts • Finger sweep		

Procedure Completed ______________________ **Date** ______________________

Notes ____

____

____

PROCEDURE

AIDING A PATIENT IN SHOCK

	Yes	No
1. Call for help.	___	___
2. Check CCCs and ABCs (Airway, Breathing, Circulation). Administer CPR if necessary.	___	___
3. Place the victim on his or her back if no spinal cord injury is suspected. Position victim so the head is lower than the rest of the body—you can place a blanket or pillow under the legs to elevate them.	___	___
4. Keep the victim warm. Cover him or her with a coat, blanket, or whatever is available.	___	___
5. Control bleeding if necessary.	___	___
6. Turn the victim's head to the side if he or she is vomiting.	___	___
7. Try to keep the environment as quiet as possible.	___	___
8. Reassure the victim and try to keep him or her calm.	___	___
9. Stay with the victim until medical help arrives.	___	___

Procedure Completed ______________________ **Date** ______________

Notes ____

____

____

PROCEDURE

AIDING A PERSON WHO SEEMS TO BE HAVING A STROKE

	Yes	No
1. Call for help.	___	___
2. Check ABCs. Administer CPR if necessary. Check blood pressure and pulse.	___	___
3. Turn the victim's head to one side so fluids can drain from the mouth.	___	___
4. If the victim is experiencing paralysis on one side, turn the victim on the affected side.	___	___
5. Elevate the head without flexing the neck.	___	___
6. Loosen tight clothing.	___	___
7. Keep the victim warm.	___	___

	Yes	No
8. Keep the victim as calm as possible.	___	___
9. Stay with the patient until medical help arrives or take the patient to an emergency medical facility.	___	___

Procedure Completed ______________________ **Date** ______________

Notes ____

____

____

PROCEDURE

HELPING TO STOP A HEMORRHAGE

	Yes	No
1. Identify the location of the bleeding.	___	___
2. Put on disposable gloves, if available. In a home situation, you can use a plastic bag or other nonabsorbent material.	___	___
3. Apply direct pressure over the wound. Use a sterile dressing or the cleanest cloth available.	___	___
4. Elevate the wound above the patient's heart.	___	___
5. Call for help.	___	___
6. If blood seeps through the dressing, apply additional dressing on top of it. Never lift or remove a dressing once it is on the wound.	___	___
7. If bleeding has not stopped, locate a pressure point between the heart and the wound and apply pressure. For example, if the wound is on the thigh, place pressure on the pressure point in the groin.	___	___
8. If bleeding has still not stopped, and the bleeding is from the arm or leg, apply a tourniquet. Once a tourniquet is applied, never remove it. It must be removed by trained medical personnel.	___	___
9. Treat the patient for shock.	___	___
10. Seek immediate medical attention.	___	___

Procedure Completed ______________________ **Date** ______________

Notes ____

____

____

PROCEDURE

HELPING A PERSON HAVING A SEIZURE

	Yes	No
1. Call for help.	___	___
2. Do not leave the victim.	___	___
3. Lower the victim to the floor.	___	___
4. Do not restrain movements.	___	___
5. Do whatever is possible to protect the patient from injury. You can place a pillow or blanket under the patient's head, or cradle the head in your lap.	___	___
6. Turn the head to the side to prevent choking.	___	___
7. Loosen tight clothing.	___	___
8. Move furniture and equipment out of the way so the person does not strike it.	___	___
9. After the seizure stops, help the patient to bed.	___	___
10. Raise the side rails.	___	___
11. Make the patient comfortable and allow him or her to rest.	___	___
12. Get medical attention for the patient.	___	___
13. Report and record seizure activity, including length of seizure in minutes and seconds, body parts involved, and patient reaction.	___	___

Procedure Completed ______________________ **Date** ______________

Notes ____

PROCEDURE

HELPING A PATIENT WITH BURNS

	Yes	No
1. Call for help.	___	___
2. Remove the victim from the source of the burn (fire, smoke, flames, chemical, sun).	___	___
3. Check ABCs. Administer CPR if necessary.	___	___
4. When a patient has a first-degree burn, immerse the body part in cold water and then cover the area with a dry, sterile dressing.	___	___

	Yes	No
5. When a patient has a second-degree burn, immerse the body part in cold water and then: • Blot the part dry with a sterile cloth. • Treat for shock. • Get medical attention.	___	___
6. When a patient has a third-degree burn: • Remove clothing from the burn site to expose it. Do not remove clothing that is stuck to the burn. • Cover the burn site with a sterile cloth or a sheet to protect it from infection. • Treat for shock. • Watch for breathing difficulty. • Get immediate medical attention.	___	___
7. When a patient has a chemical burn: • Flush the burn site with large quantities of water for at least 30 minutes. • Remove surrounding clothing. • Get medical attention.	___	___
8. Give the conscious victim plenty of fluids to maintain hydration.	___	___

Procedure Completed ______________________ **Date** ______________

Notes ____

____

____

PROCEDURE

HELPING A PATIENT WHO HAS BEEN POISONED

When a victim is conscious:

	Yes	No
1. Check the patient's ABCs. Maintain a clear airway.	___	___
2. Observe the patient.	___	___
3. Check the mouth for burns and odor.	___	___
4. Question the victim and other people present to determine the poison, the quantity, the time it was taken, and the age of the victim.	___	___
5. Look for a poison container and other clues.	___	___
6. Call the Poison Control Center for help.	___	___
7. Follow the directions given to you by the Poison Control Center. They may ask you to induce vomiting, try to prevent vomiting, or give the patient water or milk.	___	___
8. Keep the patient comfortable until medical help arrives.	___	___

	Yes	No
9. Give empty poison containers to medical personnel and report your observations to the medical staff.	___	___

When a victim is unconscious:

	Yes	No
1. Check the patient's ABCs. Maintain a clear airway.	___	___
2. Place the patient on the left side in case he or she starts to vomit.	___	___
3. Look for immediate clues to determine what type of poison was taken.	___	___
4. Call the Poison Control Center for help.	___	___
5. Perform rescue breathing or CPR only upon direction from Poison Control. Some ingested poisons make it dangerous for you to perform rescue breathing.	___	___
6. Follow the directions given to you by the Poison Control Center.	___	___
7. Keep the patient comfortable until medical help arrives.	___	___

Procedure Completed ______________________________ **Date** ______________________

Notes ____

____

____

CHAPTER 8

GETTING A JOB AS A NURSING ASSISTANT

STUDY OBJECTIVES

Many types of jobs are available for trained nursing assistants. A job search should result in finding a job, but it should also help you find out what type of nursing assisting job might be best for you. A job search requires skills that help you find leads, organize your search, interview effectively, and dress appropriately for interviews.

- Many jobs are available for nursing assistants. Some examples are geriatric aide, personal care technician, hospital attendant, ward attendant, companion, home health aide, and physical therapy aide.
- Four sources of job leads are newspapers, agencies, directories, and professional associations.
- A personal data sheet should contain all the information you need to fill out any employment application you might encounter. Answer all questions on an employment application.
- A résumé should be one page or shorter and should include your name, address, job objective, educational and work experiences, and references.
- Appropriate interview dress includes clean, neat business attire.
- Five interviewing skills are: plan your appearance, be on time, communicate effectively, answer questions honestly and carefully, and follow up on the interview.

▲ KNOW YOUR TERMS

In the space provided, write the letter of the definition that best fits the numbered term.

__1. application form	a. An exchange of information among individuals, groups, or institutions.
__2. job interview	b. A recommendation for hiring from someone who is familiar with a job applicant.
__3. networking	c. A formal meeting between a job candidate and an employer.
__4. personal data sheet	d. A sheet containing personal information likely to be needed on a job application.
__5. reference	e. A summary of one's education and work experience.
__6. résumé	f. A questionnaire filled out by an applicant for a job.

▲ TEST YOUR KNOWLEDGE

Write the word(s) that best completes the statement.

1. A companion may live with a home care ____________.
2. Local newspapers run ____________ ____________ to list available jobs.
3. Employment ____________ may be a source of job leads.
4. A ____________ ____________ ____________ lists all the information needed to fill out an application and make up a résumé.
5. A ____________ ____________ is a formal meeting between a candidate and an employer.
6. A ____________ is a recommendation from someone who can vouch for your abilities or dependability.
7. ____________ and ____________ are the most important factors in personal appearance.
8. Speak ____________ in an interview.
9. Follow up on an interview by sending a ____________.
10. A ____________ ____________ is the process of looking for a job.

▲ THINK ABOUT THE ISSUES

1. Attitude toward work is an important indicator of how well you will perform a job. In your own mind, evaluate your attitude and those of your fellow students. Who do you think will be the most successful in a job?
2. Some of your peers like to dye their hair in bright colors. Do you think an interviewer would react well to green or purple hair? Why or why not?

CHAPTER 9

HEALTH AND THE HUMAN BODY

STUDY OBJECTIVES

The body structures affect each other and how the body as a whole functions. Diseases and disorders may affect body function or mind function. The five sense organs are affected by aging. Elderly people have sexual needs and should be able to express those needs in a long-term care facility.

- The four basic structures of the human body are cells, tissues, organs, and systems.
- The major organs of the body keep the body alive. Each organ has a specific purpose.
- Several common disorders that affect the major organs are cardiovascular disease, diabetes mellitus, emphysema, and hepatitis.
- The five sensory organs are the eyes (sight), ears (sound), nose (smell), skin (touch), and taste buds (taste). The five senses are essential to our safety and well-being.
- Aging lessens the ability of the sensory organs to hear, see, smell, taste, or feel things.
- Sexuality can be expressed in many ways—hugging, holding hands, making eye contact, kissing, masturbating, and so on.
- As one ages, hormone secretions generally lessen and therefore reduce sexual urgency and strength. Psychologically, elderly people may desire as much sexual contact as when they were younger, but they may not be as physically capable as they once were.
- People in long-term care facilities have a right to sexual expression, either with a partner or by themselves. Privacy should be provided and respected.

KNOW YOUR TERMS

MATCHING EXERCISE I

In the space provided, write the letter of the definition that best fits the numbered term.

__ 1. Alzheimer's disease	a. The smallest unit of living matter capable of existing independently.
__ 2. atherosclerosis	b. The organ of hearing.
__ 3. bisexuality	c. A mental state characterized by loss of a sense of time or place.
__ 4. brain	d. A sudden interruption in the blood supply to the brain; a stroke.
__ 5. brainstem	e. A mental disorder often marked by extreme sadness and lethargy.
__ 6. cell	f. A condition of the lungs characterized by destructive enlargement and change in parts of the lung, leading to difficulty in breathing.
__ 7. cerebellum	g. A hollow muscular organ that takes in blood from the veins and sends it out to the arteries.
__ 8. cerebrovascular accident (CVA)	h. A disease characterized by underproduction and use of insulin, overproduction of urine, and excessive amounts of sugar in the blood and urine.
__ 9. cerebrum	i. Inflammation of the liver.
__10. depression	j. The portion of the brain associated with intelligence and thought.
__11. diabetes mellitus	k. A chronic, incurable disease characterized by progressive mental and physical deterioration.
__12. disorientation	l. The part of the brain connected to the spinal cord; controls heart rate, respiration, and other essential body functions.
__13. ear	m. A condition in which fat deposits build up on the inner walls of the coronary artery.
__14. emphysema	n. The portion of the brain concerned with controlling muscular activity and maintaining balance.
__15. eye	o. Interest in sexual relations with both sexes.
__16. heart	p. Sexual attraction to members of the opposite sex.
__17. hepatitis	q. The organ of vision.
__18. heterosexuality	r. The organ contained within the cranium that controls thought and neural operation.

MATCHING EXERCISE II

In the space provided, write the letter of the definition that best fits the numbered term.

__ 1. homosexuality	a. High blood pressure.
__ 2. hypertension	b. An abnormal mental condition.
__ 3. liver	c. Any major body part that performs a specific function.
__ 4. lung	d. A gland of the body that secretes digestive enzymes and hormones.
__ 5. masturbation	e. The portion of the respiratory system that includes the protruding area of the face through which we breathe, and the cavity behind it.
__ 6. mental disorder	f. A group of parts and/or organs that act together to perform certain body functions.
__ 7. mental retardation	g. A neurological disorder characterized by tremors and rigidity of movement.
__ 8. myocardial infarction	h. A collection of similar cells interconnected by an intercellular substance.
__ 9. nose	i. Sexual attraction to members of the same sex.
__10. organ	j. A tendency toward either homosexuality or heterosexuality.
__11. pancreas	k. One of the two organs of respiration.
__12. Parkinson's disease	l. The organ of the body that produces important blood proteins, stores excess sugar and protein, and produces bile to aid digestion.
__13. sense	m. The outer covering of the body.
__14. sexual orientation	n. The ability to perceive a stimulus; one of five body functions that provide this ability.
__15. skin	o. Erotic self-stimulation, usually to the point of orgasm.
__16. system	p. Parts of the surface of the tongue that aid in sensing taste.
__17. taste buds	q. A sudden insufficiency in the flow of blood to the heart muscle.
__18. tissue	r. Below-average intellectual ability, present from birth or infancy.

▲ TEST YOUR KNOWLEDGE

Write the word(s) that best completes the statement.

1. The simplest living unit of the body structure is the ____________.
2. ____________ are groups of cells that work together.

3. ______________ are groups of tissue that work in a system to perform a particular body task.
4. A cerebrovascular accident happens in the ______________.
5. The five sensory organs are the ______________, ______________, ______________, ______________, and ______________ ______________.
6. The sharpness of the senses usually ______________ with age.
7. Older adults usually can hear ______________-______________ sounds more easily than ______________-______________ sounds.
8. The organ that detects hot, cold, and pressure is the ______________.
9. Self-stimulation for sexual pleasure is ______________.
10. ______________ is finding both men and women sexually attractive.

▲ THINK ABOUT THE ISSUES

1. A patient with emphysema continues to smoke. Do you think he or she should receive the best possible medical care? Why or why not?
2. Do you accept that there are various ways to express your sexuality? Why or why not?

CHAPTER 10

ANATOMY AND PHYSIOLOGY

STUDY OBJECTIVES

The cell is the basic unit of the body. All structures of the body consist of cells. The major types of tissue in the body are connective tissue, epithelial tissue, muscle tissue, and nervous tissue. Cavities are spaces within the body that hold organs. The systems of the body are groups of organs that work together to perform one or more body functions.

▲ The cell is the basic unit of the human body. It consists of a membrane, nucleus, and cytoplasm.

▲ Connective tissue, epithelial tissue, muscle tissue, and nervous tissue are the major types of tissue in the body.

▲ The major body cavities are the dorsal in the back side of the body and the ventral in the front. The dorsal cavity contains the brain and spinal cord. The ventral cavities contain the heart, lungs, liver, pancreas, stomach, intestines, and kidneys.

▲ The major body systems are the circulatory system, respiratory system, digestive system, urinary system, reproductive system, endocrine system, nervous system, musculoskeletal system, and integumentary system.

▲ The circulatory system transports blood throughout the body. The respiratory system brings oxygen to the cells and removes carbon dioxide from the lungs. The digestive system breaks down the food we eat into a usable form, and eliminates solid waste from the body. The urinary system eliminates liquid waste from the body. The reproductive system allows for reproduction of the species. The endocrine system manufactures chemicals needed for proper body functioning. The nervous system controls the body's voluntary and involuntary functions. The musculoskeletal system includes the bones, muscles, joints, tendons, and ligaments that provide a framework for and allow the body to move. The integumentary system is the body's protective covering.

KNOW YOUR TERMS

MATCHING EXERCISE I

In the space provided, write the letter of the definition that best fits the numbered term.

__ 1. adrenal gland	a. A fibrous part of a nerve cell that carries impulses away from the neuron.
__ 2. anterior lobe	b. The organ of the body that serves as a receptacle for urine.
__ 3. anus	c. Any vessel in the body through which blood flows.
__ 4. artery	d. The system of the body that breaks down food into a form usable by the cells.
__ 5. autonomic activity	e. The system of glands that secretes hormones used throughout the body.
__ 6. autonomic nervous system	f. One of two branches of nerve cells that conduct impulses toward the center of the cell.
__ 7. axon	g. The tissue that connects bones to joints.
__ 8. bladder	h. A hormone that helps promote and maintain the development of female secondary sex characteristics.
__ 9. blood	i. The major portion of the large intestine leading to the rectum.
__10. blood vessel	j. The opening at the bottom of the digestive tract through which feces is excreted.
__11. bone	k. The part of the nervous system that controls automatic body functions (for example, breathing, blood pressure, digestion, and elimination).
__12. capillary	l. The outer layer of skin.
__13. cartilage	m. One of a pair of glands located above the kidney; it is a part of the endocrine system and produces hormones that stimulate the nervous system.
__14. cavity	n. Another name for the urinary system.
__15. central nervous system	o. A vessel that carries blood from the heart through the body.
__16. chyme	p. A hole or hollow space.
__17. circulatory system	q. Any of various organ bodies that secrete material such as hormones.
__18. colon	r. Of the back.
__19. dendrite	s. Functions that happen automatically, which we do not consciously have to tell the body to perform.

__20. digestive system	t. The part of the nervous system, including the brain and spinal cord, that controls the activities of the nervous system.
__21. dorsal	u. The system of the body that transports blood throughout the body; the heart, blood, and blood vessels.
__22. endocrine system	v. The hard parts of connective tissue that make up the skeletal structure of the body.
__23. epidermis	w. The fluid that circulates through the heart, arteries, capillaries, and veins.
__24. estrogen	x. The semifluid mass of partially digested food that passes from the stomach to the duodenum.
__25. excretory system	y. The smallest blood vessel.
__26. gland	z. A section of the pituitary gland that secretes a number of important hormones.

MATCHING EXERCISE II

In the space provided, write the letter of the definition that best fits the numbered term.

__ 1. homeostasis	a. One of two organs that excrete urine into the ureter.
__ 2. hormone	b. A body tissue that can contract and provide motion.
__ 3. integumentary system	c. The system that controls and coordinates the body's voluntary and involuntary functions.
__ 4. involuntary muscle	d. The cyclical bloody discharge from the uterus in nonpregnant females.
__ 5. joint	e. The part of the nervous system, including the cranial and spinal nerves, that carries impulses between the brain and the rest of the body.
__ 6. kidney	f. One of a pair of female reproductive glands, from which ova are released.
__ 7. ligament	g. The fluid part of the blood.
__ 8. menstruation	h. Muscle controlled by reflex and not under voluntary control.
__ 9. muscle	i. A tough band of tissue that connects bones and cartilage or supports organs or other structures.
__10. musculoskeletal system	j. A substance produced by an organ of the body and circulated to other organs to affect their functioning; a synthetic version of such a substance.
__11. nervous system	k. The organ of the body that includes the skin and its appendages.
__12. neuron	l. A part of the endocrine system that secretes substances that have an impact on most bodily functions.
__13. ovary	m. A section of the pituitary gland that secretes hormones.
__14. parasympathetic nervous system	n. Involuntary contractions of the digestive system that aid in the process of digesting food.
__15. parathyroid gland	o. A female sex hormone.
__16. peripheral nervous system	p. The framework of the body consisting of bones, muscles, joints, tendons, and ligaments.
__17. peristalsis	q. A nerve cell and its appendages.
__18. pituitary gland	r. A flattened body that is part of the blood and aids in clotting.
__19. plasma	s. A state of equilibrium or balance among parts and systems of the body.
__20. platelets	t. The end portion of the lower intestine leading to the anus.

__21. posterior lobe	u. A gland in the endocrine system that controls the use of calcium in the body.
__22. progesterone	v. The cells in the blood that contain hemoglobin and carry oxygen to the tissues.
__23. rectum	w. The process of breathing.
__24. red blood cells	x. The part of the nervous system that controls bodily functions when we are relaxed.
__25. reproductive system	y. The body system involved in the production of offspring.
__26. respiration	z. A place of contact between two or more bones, usually movable.

MATCHING EXERCISE III

In the space provided, write the letter of the definition that best fits the numbered term.

__ 1. semen	a. The part of the nervous system that is activated in response to stress, anger, or danger.
__ 2. small intestine	b. A strong, fibrous, cordlike substance that connects muscles to bones and other parts.
__ 3. sperm	c. The pair of male reproductive glands contained in the scrotum.
__ 4. sympathetic nervous system	d. The part of the intestine between the stomach and the colon.
__ 5. synovial fluid	e. The gland in the endocrine system that has an impact on immune system functioning, particularly early in life.
__ 6. tendon	f. A male hormone or a synthetic version of it that is responsible for male secondary sex characteristics.
__ 7. testes	g. A fluid that lubricates joints.
__ 8. testosterone	h. Male reproductive cells ejaculated in semen.
__ 9. thymus gland	i. A female organ that contains and nourishes the fetus prior to birth.
__10. thyroid gland	j. Any of a number of blood vessels that carry blood to the heart.
__11. urinary system	k. The viscous fluid containing sperm that is ejaculated from the penis.
__12. uterus	l. Located near the front lower part of the body.
__13. vein	m. The system of the body that produces and excretes urine.
__14. ventral	n. Any muscle controlled by conscious thought.
__15. voluntary muscle	o. Blood cells lacking hemoglobin that help the body fight infection.
__16. white blood cells	p. The gland in the endocrine system that regulates body metabolism.

▲ TEST YOUR KNOWLEDGE

Write the word(s) that best completes the statement.

1. The three parts of a cell are the ____________, ____________, and ____________.
2. Two X chromosomes are in the cells of ____________.
3. ____________ tissue is found in bones, ligaments, and tendons.
4. ____________ tissue covers the body surfaces.

5. The ______________ cavity is on the back side of the body.
6. The ______________ cavity is on the front side of the body.
7. The ______________ ______________ transports blood throughout the body.
8. The excretory system is also know as the ______________ ______________.
9. The nervous system controls the body's ______________ and ______________ functions.
10. The ______________ ______________ includes the body's protective covering.

▲ THINK ABOUT THE ISSUES

1. Every year, more organ transplants are performed. What do you think about organ donation? Do you plan to be an organ donor? Why or why not?
2. What do you think is the body's most important organ?

CHAPTER 11

STANDARD PRECAUTIONS: INFECTION, DISEASE, AND DISABILITY

STUDY OBJECTIVES

Diseases are either infectious (spreadable) or noninfectious (unable to be spread). Standard precautions help prevent the spread of infection. Certain diseases and disabilities usually require long-term care. Your own personal wellness is important to you and your patients.

- Infectious diseases are caused by harmful microorgansims. These diseases can be spread from one person to another. Noninfectious diseases have a variety of causes, and cannot be spread from one person to another.
- AIDS is a major infectious disease found in patients in long-term care facilities.
- Standard precautions include handwashing, gloving, gowning, and masking.
- Noninfectious diseases that often require long-term care are Alzheimer's disease, stroke, and heart disease.
- Major patient disabilities include hemiplegia, paraplegia, and quadriplegia. Some of these result in loss of bowel or bladder control.
- Personal wellness means maintaining good health and following all safety precautions and procedures to protect yourself from injury and infection.

KNOW YOUR TERMS

MATCHING EXERCISE 1

In the space provided, write the letter of the definition that best fits the numbered term.

__ 1. airborne transmission	a. A group of yeast or mold organisms, especially ones that affect skin or nails.
__ 2. animal (vectorborne) transmission	b. Transmission of a disease that occurs when one human touches another person or the excretions of another person who is infected with certain diseases.
__ 3. asepsis	c. The system of the body that fights disease.
__ 4. autoclave	d. A state of sterility; a state where no harmful microorganisms are present.
__ 5. bacteria	e. A device used to sterilize implements.
__ 6. Centers for Disease Control and Prevention (CDC)	f. Transmission of a disease that occurs when microorganisms are transferred from one person to another in droplets passed through coughing, sneezing, and talking.
__ 7. common vehicle transmission	g. A division of the U.S. Public Health Service that researches diseases and develops standards and methods for controlling them.
__ 8. contaminated	h. Transmission of a disease that occurs when a person ingests or touches something contaminated with microorganisms.
__ 9. direct contact	i. A disease capable of being transmitted by infection.
__10. disinfection	j. Soiled or polluted (especially with harmful microorganisms).
__11. droplet transmission	k. An environment that allows microorganisms to grow.
__12. fungus	l. The process of cleaning so as to remove harmful microorganisms.
__13. hemiplegia	m. A nosocomial infection that is resistant to currently available antibiotics.
__14. host	n. A group of procedures and guidelines for separating patients, used to prevent the spread of infection.
__15. immune system	o. Transmission of a disease via microorganisms carried through the air.
__16. infectious disease	p. Transmission of disease that occurs when an animal bites a human.
__17. isolation techniques	q. Total or partial paralysis of one side of the body.
__18. methicillin resistant Staphylococcus aureus (MRSA)	r. One-celled microorganism.

MATCHING EXERCISE II

In the space provided, write the letter of the definition that best fits the numbered term.

Term	Definition
__ 1. microorganism	a. An infection gotten from a hospital environment.
__ 2. mycotic	b. Paralysis of all four limbs.
__ 3. noninfectious disease	c. A harmful microorganism.
__ 4. nonpathogen	d. Paralysis of the lower half of the body.
__ 5. nosocomial infection	e. Bacteria covered with a hard shell.
__ 6. Occupational Safety and Health Administration (OSHA)	f. One-celled parasitic microorganisms.
__ 7. paraplegia	g. An environment in which microorganisms (especially harmful ones) can grow.
__ 8. pathogen	h. Free of harmful microorganisms; pure.
__ 9. protozoa	i. The smallest type of microorganism, usually causing disease and that is spread from one person to another.
__10. Pseudomonas aeruginosa	j. A helpful microorganism.
__11. quadriplegia	k. A nosocomial infection that is difficult to control with current antibiotics.
__12. reservoir	l. A poisonous substance.
__13. salmonella	m. Afflicted with a fungus (as a toenail).
__14. spores	n. A disease that cannot be passed from one person to another.
__15. toxin	o. A group of bacteria (usually found in contaminated food) that causes illness.
__16. uncontaminated	p. A nosocomial infection that is resistant to currently available antibiotics.
__17. vancomycin resistant enterococci (VRE)	q. A division of the U.S. Department of Labor that enforces standards for safety and health programs on the job.
__18. virus	r. A microscopic organism.

▲ TEST YOUR KNOWLEDGE

Write the word(s) that best completes the statement.

1. Harmful microorganisms are called ____________.
2. A ____________ or host is an environment in which microorganisms can grow.
3. The common cold is caused by a ____________, the smallest type of microorganism.
4. ____________ transmission occurs when microorganisms travel in the air and are then inhaled by the host.

5. A person with a strong ______________ ______________ usually has the ability to fight disease.
6. The absence of pathogens is ______________.
7. An ______________ disease can spread from one person to another.
8. ______________ results when the body cannot produce enough insulin.
9. A ______________ ______________ is another name for a heart attack.
10. A patient with ______________ is paralyzed from the neck down.

THINK ABOUT THE ISSUES

1. Many families try to care for patients with Alzheimer's disease at home. How do you think your family would deal with a family member with Alzheimer's disease?
2. Health care work can be dangerous if you do not follow standard precautions and safety rules. If you knew a fellow worker was acting irresponsibly about health precautions, what would you do? How dangerous is it for you if someone you are working with does not follow standard precautions?

CHAPTER 12

MEDICAL TERMINOLOGY

STUDY OBJECTIVES

The special language of health care is called medical terminology. Medical terms are usually made up of parts—prefixes, combining forms, and suffixes. Abbreviations are used, especially in patient records or doctors' notes. Medical specialties are the areas of concentration for doctors.

- ▲ Prefixes, combining forms, and suffixes make up medical terms.
- ▲ Medical prefixes often define a direction, such as away from or toward. Combining forms may represent body parts or conditions. Suffixes often refer to something that happens or is done, such as removal or cutting.
- ▲ Abbreviations used in health care include measurements, orders, conditions, time, and titles.
- ▲ Common medical specialists include the surgeon, obstetrician, pediatrician, oncologist, psychiatrist, and so on.
- ▲ Medical symbols are used in charts, prescriptions, for safety, and for identification.

▲ KNOW YOUR TERMS

In the space provided, write the letter of the definition that best fits the numbered term.

__ 1. abbreviation	a. An element placed at the end of a word.
__ 2. combining form	b. A basic word element that has meaning.
__ 3. prefix	c. A field of medical practice in which a practitioner concentrates.
__ 4. root	d. A root with a combining vowel that forms words when put together with other word parts.
__ 5. specialty	e. An element placed at the beginning of a word.
__ 6. suffix	f. A shortened form of a word or phrase.
__ 7. symbol	g. A written or printed sign that has specific meaning.

▲ TEST YOUR KNOWLEDGE

Write the word(s) that best completes the statement.

1. Elements at the beginnings of words are ____________.
2. Basic word elements that have meaning are ____________.
3. The special language of a profession is known as ____________.
4. The prefix anti- means ____________.
5. The combining form laryngo- means ____________.
6. A suffix is an element that attaches at the ____________ of words.
7. The suffix ____________ means pain.
8. DNR is an abbreviation for ____________ ____________ ____________.
9. A pediatrician treats ____________.
10. The symbol > means ____________ ____________.

▲ THINK ABOUT THE ISSUES

Do you think learning a jargon is important? Why or why not?

CHAPTER 13

COMMUNICATION IN THE FACILITY—OBSERVING, CHARTING, AND REPORTING

STUDY OBJECTIVES

Communication in the facility is part of the nursing assistant's job. Nursing assistants must relate well to patients and to other members of the staff. The observations they make, chart, and report must be accurate and clear. Most facilities have rules for maintaining patient records. Some use computers to aid in keeping records.

- Nursing assistants observe residents by gathering objective information using their own senses and by gathering subjective information (what the patient or others tell you about the patient's condition).
- The guidelines for effective communication are careful listening; observing of nonverbal communication; speaking clearly and pleasantly; precise reporting.
- Nursing assistants make reports by writing down observations in records, by tape-recording observations, or by giving verbal descriptions to a staff member.
- Patient records are usually maintained in written form in a file or chart. The record usually contains a graphic chart, a daily flow sheet, and nurses' notes.
- Many health care facilities are changing over to computerized records, which enable information to be available to many people at the same time.

KNOW YOUR TERMS

In the space provided, write the letter of the definition that best fits the numbered term.

__ 1. body language	a. Nurses' written information about a patient's condition.
__ 2. charting	b. A patient's chart that records observations and vital signs measurements.
__ 3. flow sheet	c. Any spoken or written communication.
__ 4. graphic chart	d. Something that can be perceived and usually recorded.
__ 5. interpersonal skills	e. The process of describing observations and care given.
__ 6. message	f. The person who sends a message.
__ 7. nurses' notes	g. A written or computerized record of the care and observations of a patient.
__ 8. nursing care plan	h. Entering data into a patient's record.
__ 9. objective information	i. Information that is a matter of opinion and not the result of observable events.
__10. observation	j. The person to whom a communication is sent.
__11. patient record	k. Information that can be seen or verified.
__12. receiver	l. Abilities that enable one person to relate to another effectively.
__13. recording	m. The mannerisms and gestures used in communication.
__14. reporting	n. A chart used to record data (as the intake and output of a patient).
__15. sender	o. The putting of medical and related facts into a patient's record.
__16. subjective information	p. A document written by a nurse that outlines the care to be given to a specific individual.

TEST YOUR KNOWLEDGE

Write the word(s) that best completes the statement.

1. A sign or symptom you see or measure is part of ______________ information.
2. A sign or symptom you hear about is part of ______________ information.
3. In communication, one person is the ______________ of a message and the other person is the ______________.
4. The ______________ ______________ ______________ report keeps the incoming shift up-to-date on each patient's condition.
5. Recording is also referred to as ______________.

6. A ______________ ______________ ______________ details the care required for a patient.
7. A medical chart is a ______________ document.
8. A resident's ADLs are usually recorded on a ______________ ______________.
9. The observations and measurements of a patient's physical condition are usually recorded on a ______________ ______________
10. ______________ is a type of patient card file system.

THINK ABOUT THE ISSUES

1. Discuss some of the possible legal uses for a patient's chart.
2. Computers are very convenient because they can keep mass amounts of information readily available. What are some of the privacy issues that might be a problem when patient records are kept on computers?

CHAPTER 14

Care of the Resident's Room

Study Objectives

Nursing assistants take care of residents' rooms, making sure they are clean, pleasant, and safe. This constitutes a major task of nursing assisting. Cleanliness helps avoid the spread of infection. A pleasant environment helps maintain the resident's well-being.

- ▲ A safe resident environment includes a well-lit, well-ventilated room kept at comfortable temperatures. Floors must not be slippery and pathways must be kept clear.
- ▲ A pleasant room with reminders of the past and of family life help a resident stay connected to the activities they once loved and the people they care about. This connection helps maintain their psychological well-being.
- ▲ Residents' rooms typically have a bed, chair, a bedside stand, a wastebasket, personal hygiene items, personal mementos, a closet with clothing, and a privacy curtain or screen.
- ▲ Wash hands before handling clean linens and after handling soiled linens. Always put clean linens on a clean surface. Never shake linens or allow them to come in contact with your uniform. Dispose of dirty linens properly.
- ▲ When making beds, do one side of the bed first, then work on the other side. Beds are made according to their use. A closed bed is not currently in use. An open bed is a bed used by an ambulatory resident. An occupied bed is used by a patient who is bedridden.

▲ KNOW YOUR TERMS

In the space provided, write the letter of the definition that best fits the numbered term.

__ 1. closed bed

__ 2. drawsheet

__ 3. occupied bed

__ 4. open bed

__ 5. surgical bed

__ 6. toe tuck

__ 7. unoccupied bed

a. A bed that must be made while the resident remains in it.

b. A bed that is used by a resident who gets up during the day.

c. A bed made so that it allows easy transfer from a stretcher to a bed (as for a patient returning from surgery).

d. The tucking of the top bed linens under the bottom end of a mattress loosely, so as to leave enough room for the resident to move feet and toes comfortably.

e. A bed in a health care facility not currently in use.

f. Another name for open bed.

g. A small sheet placed over a bottom sheet in bedmaking.

▲ TEST YOUR KNOWLEDGE

Write the word(s) that best completes the statement.

1. Temperatures in a cold climate usually need to be ____________ more for elderly people than for younger people.
2. There is a greater likelihood of accidents in a room that is not ____________.
3. Each resident's room usually includes some ____________ ____________ kept as mementos of their families and friends.
4. Wash hands ____________ handling ____________ linens.
5. Wash hands ____________ handling ____________ linens.
6. A ____________ bed is one that is not being used by a resident or patient.
7. An ____________ bed is one used by an ambulatory resident or patient.
8. An ____________ bed is one used by a patient who is bedridden.
9. A ____________ bed is one made up for someone returning from surgery.
10. A ____________ ____________ leaves the top linens loose so the patient can freely move his or her feet or toes.

THINK ABOUT THE ISSUES

1. Many facilities have rules about the type and quantity of personal belongings allowed in each resident's room. Why do you think they have such rules?
2. Residents often take naps or just rest during the day. They may unmake a bed several times during the day. What should your attitude be about having to remake the bed several times?

CHECK YOUR SKILLS

In the following procedure checklists, check each task box that applies and answer yes or no to each step you have completed. If possible, have your instructor sign off when you have completed a procedure.

PROCEDURE

OBRA

MAKING A CLOSED BED

Standard Precautions ☐ Handwashing ☐ Gloving ☐ Gowning ☐ Masking

Introductory Tasks ☐ Gather Equipment ☐ Identify/Introduce/Explain ☐ Provide Privacy

Step	Yes	No
3. Arrange the linens in the order you put them on the bed. The items needed first should be on top, and items needed last on the bottom.	___	___
4. If possible, raise or lower the bed so it is at a comfortable working height.	___	___
5. Slide the mattress forward toward the head of the bed until it reaches the headboard.	___	___
6. If facility policy is to use a mattress pad, place the pad on the mattress, even with the top of the mattress.	___	___
7. Place the bottom sheet, sewn side down, on the mattress and unfold it lengthwise. **a.** Align the center crease in the sheet with the center of the mattress. **b.** Place the lower edge of the sheet so it lines up with the bottom of the mattress.	___	___
8. Open the bottom sheet. Make sure that about the same length of sheet hangs over each side.	___	___
9. Check to make sure that about 12 to 18 inches of sheet is available to tuck under each side.	___	___
10. At the head of the bed, lift the mattress slightly and tuck the top of the sheet under the mattress.	___	___
11. Make a mitered corner at the head of the bed. Tuck the sheet underneath the mattress along the sides of the bed. Work on one side of the bed until it is complete before working on the other side.	___	___

	Yes	No
12. Place a pad, a plastic drawsheet, or other moisture-resistant product on the mattress about 14 inches from the head of the bed pad. (Some residents do not need any pad. Follow your supervisor's instructions.)	___	___
13. Open the plastic drawsheet and tuck it under the mattress.	___	___
14. Place the cotton drawsheet over the pad or plastic drawsheet to completely cover the plastic sheet.	___	___
15. Open the cotton drawsheet and tuck it under the mattress.	___	___
16. Place the top sheet on the mattress and unfold it lengthwise. **a.** Check to be sure the stitching on the hem is facing upward, away from the patient's skin. **b.** Align the top of the sheet with the head of the mattress. **c.** Align the center crease in the sheet with the center of the mattress.	___	___
17. Place the blanket on the bed and unfold it. **a.** Align the center crease in the blanket with the center of the mattress. **b.** Place the top hem of the blanket about 6 to 8 inches from the head of the mattress.	___	___
18. Place the bedspread on the bed and unfold it. **a.** Align the center crease in the bedspread with the center of the mattress. **b.** Align the top of the bedspread with the head of the mattress. **c.** Check that the side of the bedspread facing the door is even and covers all the bed linens.	___	___
19. Tuck the top linens in together at the foot of the bed. Make a mitered corner on both sides. Check that the bed linens are smooth and tight.	___	___
20. Turn the top of the bedspread down over the blanket to make a cuff.	___	___
21. Turn the top sheet down over the bedspread.	___	___
22. Lay the pillows on the bed.	___	___
23. Open each pillowcase and lay it flat on the bed.	___	___
24. Place the pillow inside the pillowcase. Fold the corners of the seam end of the pillow inward to make a "V," open the pillowcase, slide the "V" end of the pillow into the pillowcase, and then flatten out the corners.	___	___
25. Place the pillow at the head of the bed, with the open end facing away from the door. Fold the extra pillowcase material under the pillow.	___	___
26. Pull the bedspread up over the pillows.	___	___
27. Lower the bed to its lowest possible position.	___	___
28. Place the signal light near the head of the bed.	___	___
29. Check to make sure the bed and room look neat and clean.	___	___
30. Wash your hands.	___	___

Procedure Completed ______________________ **Date** ______________

Notes ____

____

____

PROCEDURE

OBRA

MAKING AN OPEN BED

Standard Precautions ☐ Handwashing ☐ Gloving ☐ Gowning ☐ Masking

Introductory Tasks ☐ Gather Equipment ☐ Identify/Introduce/Explain ☐ Provide Privacy

	Yes	No
3. Make a closed bed (follow Steps 1 through 17 of Procedure, Making a Closed Bed). (Note that if the bed is soiled, wear disposable gloves while removing the soiled linens. Discard the gloves and wash your hands before handling the clean linens.)	___	___
4. Grasp the top cuff of the bedding in both hands.	___	___
5. Fanfold the bed linens to the foot of the bed.	___	___
6. Place the signal light near the head of the bed.	___	___
7. Lower the bed to its lowest position.	___	___
8. Wash your hands.	___	___

Procedure Completed ______________________ **Date** ______________

Notes ____

____

____

PROCEDURE

OBRA

MAKING AN OCCUPIED BED

Standard Precautions ☐ Handwashing ☐ Gloving ☐ Gowning ☐ Masking

Introductory Tasks ☐ Gather Equipment ☐ Identify/Introduce/Explain ☐ Provide Privacy

	Yes	No
7. Remove the signal light from the bed.	___	___
8. Raise or lower the bed if possible to achieve a comfortable working position.	___	___
9. Lower the head of the bed as flat as possible for patient comfort and safety.	___	___
10. Lower the side rail on the side of the bed that is closest to you. The other side rail should be in the upright position and locked.	___	___

	Yes	No
11. Loosen the top bed linens at the foot of the bed.	___	___
12. Take off the bedspread. Fold it neatly if it will be reused.	___	___
13. Take off the blanket. Fold it neatly if it is to be reused.	___	___
14. Place a bath blanket over the top sheet, if it is still covering the patient.	___	___
15. Ask the patient to hold the top edge of the bath blanket. If he or she cannot, tuck the blanket under both shoulders.	___	___
16. Gently reach under the bath blanket and pull the top sheet down toward the foot of the bed. When it reaches the foot of the bed, remove the sheet from the bed, and place in the hamper or laundry bag.	___	___
17. Slide the mattress to the head of the bed.	___	___
18. Ask the patient to turn onto his or her side, facing away from you. If necessary, help the patient turn in bed. The patient should be positioned on the far side of the bed in proper body alignment (see Chapter 16).	___	___
19. Move the pillow to the far side of the bed and place it under the patient's head. Adjust it for the patient's comfort.	___	___
20. Loosen the bottom bed linens, starting at the head of the bed and working towards the foot.	___	___
21. Fanfold the bottom bed linens toward the patient, one at a time.	___	___
22. If the mattress pad will be replaced, fanfold it also. If it will be reused, straighten it.	___	___
23. If appropriate, place a clean mattress pad on the bed. **a.** Unfold it lengthwise. **b.** Make sure the center crease in the pad aligns with the center of the mattress. **c.** Fanfold half of the pad toward the patient.	___	___
24. Place a clean bottom sheet on top of the pad. **a.** Unfold it lengthwise. **b.** Make sure the center crease in the sheet aligns with the center of the mattress. **c.** Make sure the stitching on the hem is facing away from the patient. **d.** Check to see that the hem is even with the bottom of the mattress. **e.** Fanfold the sheet toward the patient.	___	___
25. Make a mitered corner at the head of the bed.	___	___
26. Tuck the sheet underneath the mattress along the side of the bed closest to you.	___	___
27. Place the plastic drawsheet on the bed, about 14 inches from the head of the bed. **a.** Fanfold half of the plastic drawsheet toward the patient. **b.** Tuck in the excess under the mattress.	___	___
28. Place the cotton drawsheet so that it covers the entire plastic drawsheet. **a.** Fanfold half of the cotton drawsheet toward the patient. **b.** Tuck in the excess under the mattress.	___	___
29. Raise the side rail on the side of the bed closest to you. Lock it in the upright position.	___	___
30. Walk to the other side of the bed and lower the side rail.	___	___

	Yes	No
31. Ask the patient to turn onto his or her other side. If necessary, help the patient turn in bed. The patient should be positioned on the side of the bed away from you, in proper body alignment.	___	___
32. Remove the soiled pillowcase and place a clean one over the pillow.	___	___
33. Raise the patient's head and adjust the pillow to a comfortable position.	___	___
34. Remove the soiled bottom bed linens from the bed and place in the hamper or laundry bag.	___	___
35. Straighten out the mattress pad.	___	___
36. Grasp the clean bottom sheet and pull it toward you. **a.** Make a mitered corner at the head of the bed. **b.** Tuck the sheet in along the side.	___	___
37. Bring the plastic and cotton drawsheets toward you. Tuck both drawsheets under the mattress.	___	___
38. Ask the patient to lie on his or her back in the middle of the mattress. Assist the patient if necessary. Arrange the pillow in a comfortable position for the patient.	___	___
39. Place the clean top sheet on the bed. **a.** Unfold it lengthwise. **b.** Make sure the center crease in the sheet aligns with the center of the mattress. **c.** Make sure the stitching on the hem is facing away from the patient. **d.** Check to see that the hem is even with the head of the mattress.	___	___
40. Ask the patient to hold the top sheet. If he or she cannot, tuck it under both shoulders.	___	___
41. Gently remove the bath blanket.	___	___
42. Place the blanket on the bed. **a.** Unfold it lengthwise. **b.** Make sure the center crease in the blanket aligns with the center of the mattress. **c.** Make sure the upper hem of the blanket is 6 to 8 inches from the head of the bed.	___	___
43. Place the bedspread on the bed. **a.** Unfold it lengthwise. **b.** Make sure the center crease in the bedspread aligns with the center of the mattress. **c.** Make sure the upper hem of the bedspread lines up with the top of the mattress.	___	___
44. Turn the top 18 inches of the bedspread down over the blanket to form a cuff.	___	___
45. Turn the top sheet down over the bedspread to make a cuff.	___	___
46. Go to the foot of the bed and lift the mattress using one arm.	___	___
47. With the other arm, tuck all the top bed linens under the mattress on that side. Leave the top linens loose enough to allow the patient to freely move his or her feet and toes. This is known as a **toe tuck**. Make a mitered corner.	___	___
48. Raise the side rail on the side of the bed where you just finished working. Lock it in the upright position.	___	___
49. Move to the other side of the bed and lower the side rail.	___	___
50. Straighten the top bed linens and tuck them in as you did on the other side of the bed. Make a mitered corner. Make a toe tuck to allow room for the toes.	___	___

	Yes	No
51. Place the signal light in a position the patient can easily reach.	___	___
52. Raise the side rail and lock it.	___	___
53. Raise the head of the bed to a position that is comfortable for the patient.	___	___
54. Lower the bed to its lowest possible position.	___	___
55. Open the curtain.	___	___
56. Wash your hands.	___	___

Procedure Completed ______________________ **Date** ______________________

Notes ____

____

____

PROCEDURE

MAKING A SURGICAL BED

Standard Precautions ☐ Handwashing ☐ Gloving ☐ Gowning ☐ Masking

Introductory Tasks ☐ Gather Equipment ☐ Identify/Introduce/Explain ☐ Provide Privacy

	Yes	No
3. Arrange the linens in the order you put them on the bed. The items needed first should be on top, and items needed last on the bottom.	___	___
4. Raise or lower the bed so it is at a comfortable working height.	___	___
5. Remove the signal light from the bed.	___	___
6. Remove linens from the bed. Place soiled bed linens in the hamper or laundry bag.	___	___
7. Follow procedure for making a closed bed. Do not tuck the top bed linens under the mattress.	___	___
8. Fold the bottom of the top bed linens back up onto the bed. The fold at the foot of the bed should be even with the edge of the mattress.	___	___
9. Fanfold the bedspread, blanket, and top sheet to the far side of the bed.	___	___
10. Place a clean pillowcase on the pillow.	___	___
11. Place the pillow upright against the headboard.	___	___
12. Raise the bed to stretcher height.	___	___
13. Be sure that all side rails are down.	___	___
14. Put the box of tissues and the emesis basin on top of the bedside stand.	___	___

	Yes	No
15. Move any furniture that would be in the way of the stretcher.	___	___
16. Wash your hands.	___	___

Procedure Completed ________________________ **Date** ____________________

Notes ____

____

____

CHAPTER 15

ADMISSION, TRANSFER, AND DISCHARGE

STUDY OBJECTIVES

Admission, transfer, and discharge of patients are often stressful times for families and patients. During admissions, patients enter a facility, give information to the staff, and are brought to their floor where they meet staff, roommates, and neighbors. Patients can transfer within a facility or to another facility. Patients are usually discharged to an independent living situation.

- During admissions, residents are introduced into a facility. A clerk usually gathers information for the patient's record. The nursing assistant may introduce the new resident to the staff and residents on the floor, show the resident around the floor, help the resident get settled, explain procedures, take vital signs, and record and report observations.
- When residents transfer, nursing assistants help them get dressed, pack up, and say good-bye. They then take them to the new unit or to a vehicle for transfer.
- During discharge, nursing assistants make sure all items are packed. They usually escort the resident out of the facility.

KNOW YOUR TERMS

In the space provided, write the letter of the definition that best fits the numbered term.

__ 1. admission	a. To release from a facility.
__ 2. dietitian	b. To move from one part of a facility to another or from one facility to another.
__ 3. discharge	c. A specialist who formulates diets based on nutrition and on medical need.
__ 4. transfer	d. The process of bringing patients or residents into a health care facility, registering them, and settling them into their rooms.

TEST YOUR KNOWLEDGE

Write the word(s) that best completes the statement.

1. ______________ is the official entry of a person into a health care facility.
2. An ______________ ______________ includes basic information about the new patient.
3. Learning how to operate the ______________ ______________ is important for new patients.
4. A ______________ occurs when a resident is moved from one unit or room to another.
5. Moving a patient from one facility to another is called a ______________.
6. Many transfers occur because of changes in a patient's ______________ condition.
7. A ______________ is a patient's authorized release from a health care facility.
8. The patient's discharge instructions include information about ______________ treatments.
9. The patient's discharge instructions also include dietary plans usually prepared by a ______________.
10. Many communities have ______________ agencies that can provide assistance after discharge from a facility.

THINK ABOUT THE ISSUES

1. Many people find change difficult. What are some of the reasons why patients might find admission, transfer, or discharge difficult?
2. Referral agencies often have support groups for people with specific illnesses. How do you think a support group might help?

CHECK YOUR SKILLS

In the following procedure checklists, check each task box that applies and answer yes or no to each step you have completed. If possible, have your instructor sign off when you have completed a procedure.

PROCEDURE

PREPARING A ROOM FOR A NEW ADMISSION

Standard Precautions ☐ Handwashing ☐ Gloving ☐ Gowning ☐ Masking

Introductory Tasks ☐ Gather Equipment ☐ Identify/Introduce/Explain ☐ Provide Privacy

	Yes	No
2. Open the bed. Fanfold the linens to the bottom of the bed.	___	___
3. Neatly fold the gown or pajamas and place them at the foot of the bed.	___	___
4. Unpack the patient pack and place the contents in the bedside table.	___	___
5. Arrange the admissions checklist, clothing list, and valuables envelope on the overbed table. For hospital admissions, also collect a sphygmomanometer, stethoscope, thermometer, and specimen container.	___	___
6. Lower the bed if the patient is ambulatory or arriving by wheelchair. Raise the bed if the patient is arriving by stretcher.	___	___
7. Clip the signal cord to the linens at the top of the bed.	___	___
8. Wash your hands.	___	___
9. Report to the supervisor that the room is ready for the patient.	___	___

Procedure Completed ______________________ **Date** ______________

Notes ____

____

____

PROCEDURE

ADMITTING A NEW PATIENT

Standard Precautions ☐ Handwashing ☐ Gloving ☐ Gowning ☐ Masking

Introductory Tasks ☐ Gather Equipment ☐ Identify/Introduce/Explain ☐ Provide Privacy

	Yes	No
6. For a hospital admission, help the patient undress and put on the gown or pajamas. Help the long-term care facility resident into comfortable clothing.	___	___
7. Make the patient comfortable in bed or on a chair.	___	___

	Yes	No
8. Put away the patient's street clothes. Complete the clothing list or inventory slip. Put the clothes in the closet or pack them for the family to take home.	___	___
9. Place the patient's valuables in the valuables envelope. Complete the form according to policy. The patient may choose to keep a small amount of money in the bedside table.	___	___
10. Place personal items in the bedside table.	___	___
11. Take any medications the patient has brought from home and bring them to the nurse when you complete the admissions process.	___	___
12. Complete the procedures needed on the admissions checklist, according to facility policy. These may include: weight, height, vital signs.	___	___
13. If a urine sample is required, describe the procedure for collecting urine. Assist the patient to the bathroom or provide a urinal or bedpan. If you assist the patient to the bathroom, point out the signal cord and other safety measures. Practice standard precautions when in contact with urine and other body fluids. Label the specimen according to facility policy.	___	___
14. Assist the patient back to the bed or chair.	___	___
15. If the patient is allowed to have water, fill the water pitcher and place it within the patient's reach. Some patients entering a hospital have NPO orders, which means they may have no food or fluids by mouth.	___	___
16. Orient the patient to the new environment by explaining: • How to operate the signal cord • How to operate the bed • The contents of the bedside table and how each item is used • How to use the television and radio • How to operate the lights • How to use the telephone • When meals are served and how to fill out a menu • Visiting hours • Names of the nursing team members • Location of the chapel, library, dining room, and other places the patient may visit	___	___
17. Ask the patient if there are any questions.	___	___
18. Complete the admissions checklist.	___	___
19. Unscreen the patient if the patient had requested privacy.	___	___
20. Deliver the urine specimen, medications, clothing list, valuables envelope, and admissions checklist to the nurse's station.	___	___
21. Wash your hands.	___	___
22. Invite family members and visitors back in the room if they were asked to leave earlier. Explain visiting hours and policies.	___	___
23. Ask the patient if anything else if needed.	___	___
24. Before leaving the room, make sure the room is neat, the signal cord is within reach of the patient, and the patient is comfortable.	___	___
25. Report your observations to the nurse.	___	___

Procedure Completed ______________________ Date ______________

Notes ____

____

____

PROCEDURE

OBRA SP

TRANSFERRING A PATIENT

Standard Precautions ☐ Handwashing ☐ Gloving ☐ Gowning ☐ Masking

Introductory Tasks ☐ Gather Equipment ☐ Identify/Introduce/Explain ☐ Provide Privacy

	Yes	No
6. Collect the patient's personal belongings. Place them in the patient's luggage or in the transfer bag. Place the luggage or bag on the bed, cart, or patient's lap to ensure items are not lost.	___	___
7. Physically transfer the patient.	___	___
8. By wheelchair: Assist the patient into the wheelchair and wheel him or her to the new room/location.	___	___
9. By stretcher or bed: Get someone to help you move the patient onto a stretcher. Raise the side rails of the stretcher or bed and fasten the safety straps for transport. Push it to the new room/location.	___	___
10. Introduce the patient to the nursing staff. Deliver the patient's chart to the charge nurse (done by the nurse in some facilities).	___	___
11. Introduce the patient to the roommate.	___	___
12. If the patient prefers privacy while getting settled, provide for privacy.	___	___
13. Make the patient comfortable in the bed or chair.	___	___
14. Bring the belongings to the new room. Place the clothes in the closet and personal items in the bedside table.	___	___
15. Unscreen the patient if the patient had requested privacy.	___	___
16. Ask the patient if he or she needs anything else.	___	___
17. Wash your hands.	___	___
18. Report the following to the receiving nurse: • The patient is in the new unit • How the patient tolerated the transfer • Any observations of the patient during the transfer	___	___
19. Return to your unit. Report the following to the nurse: • The patient has been transferred • The time of the transfer	___	___

	Yes	No
• How the patient tolerated the transfer • Any observations of the patient during the transfer		
20. Follow your facility's procedure for cleaning the room the patient has vacated.	___	___
21. Wash your hands.	___	___

Procedure Completed ______________________ **Date** ______________________

Notes ____

____

____

PROCEDURE

DISCHARGING A PATIENT

Standard Precautions ☐ Handwashing ☐ Gloving ☐ Gowning ☐ Masking

Introductory Tasks ☐ Gather Equipment ☐ Identify/Introduce/Explain ☐ Provide Privacy

	Yes	No
6. Help the patient dress.	___	___
7. Help the patient collect all personal belongings. Check the clothes against the clothing list that was completed when the patient was admitted. Have the patient sign the list to indicate that all clothing has been returned. Family members are often involved in helping the patient prepare to leave the facility.	___	___
8. Pack the patient's personal belongings. Check drawers, closet, bedside table, and bathroom for belongings.	___	___
9. Return valuables according to facility policy. Check the valuables against the inventory made at the time of admission.	___	___
10. Tell the nurse that the patient is ready for the discharge interview. The nurse will give the patient discharge instructions and prescriptions for medications.	___	___
11. Bring a wheelchair or stretcher to the patient. Lock the wheelchair. Assist the patient into the wheelchair or onto the stretcher.	___	___
12. Place the patient's luggage on the cart or give it to a family member.	___	___
13. Carry out the discharge procedure according to the facility. Patients may be required to visit the business office or discharge desk before leaving. Make sure the charge nurse or the business office removes the ID bracelet if one was given at admission. Give the discharge paperwork to the patient according to facility policy.	___	___
14. Take the patient to the front entrance. Have a coworker follow with the luggage.	___	___

	Yes	No
Remember, the patient is the facility's responsibility until he or she leaves the facility. The patient must be safely escorted out of the building to whomever is waiting.		
15. Lock the wheelchair. Assist the patient from the wheelchair or stretcher and into the car, ambulette, or ambulance.	___	___
16. Place the patient's luggage in the transport vehicle.	___	___
17. Say good-bye to the patient and close the vehicle door.	___	___
18. Return the wheelchair or stretcher to the unit. Clean and return the equipment.	___	___
19. Wash your hands.	___	___
20. Return to the patient's room. Strip the bed and place the linen in the dirty linen hamper.	___	___
21. Notify the housekeeping department that the room is ready to be cleaned.	___	___
22. Wash your hands.	___	___
23. Bring the paperwork to the nurse according to facility policy. Report the following: • The patient has been discharged • Time of discharge • Transportation used for discharge (wheelchair, stretcher) • Who accompanied the patient (parent, child, spouse, friend) • How the patient tolerated the procedure • Your observations of anything unusual	___	___

Procedure Completed ______________________ **Date** ______________________

Notes ____

____

____

CHAPTER 16

BODY MECHANICS

STUDY OBJECTIVES

Using proper body mechanics helps avoid injury to nursing assistants and to patients. Moving a patient in and out of bed and positioning patients require proper body mechanics. Transfer belts are used for safety. Mechanical lifts are used for patients who are unable to assist. Positioning, transferring, and range-of-motion exercises help keep patients comfortable.

- ▲ Body mechanics is the use of the body to lift and move. Maintaining proper alignment and good posture helps avoid back strain.
- ▲ Transferring patients to a chair or wheelchair can be done by one or two nursing assistants. Make sure to use a transfer belt when moving patients out of or into bed.
- ▲ When a patient is able to assist you while moving up in bed, have the patient push off with his or her feet to make your task easier.
- ▲ To move a helpless patient up in bed, have a team member assist you and use proper body mechanics.
- ▲ Helping a patient sit and dangle means getting the patient to a sitting position and positioning the legs.
- ▲ There are several methods for turning or rolling a patient. One is to use a drawsheet; another is to ask a team member to help you.
- ▲ Patients need to be positioned for physical comfort or for an examination. They should be draped or covered appropriately.
- ▲ A transfer belt is a safety device used in helping patients walk or moving patients into and out of bed.
- ▲ The procedure for transferring a patient to a chair or wheelchair includes the use of good body mechanics, a transfer belt, and helping the patient maintain balance.
- ▲ Mechanical lifts are used to move patients who are bedridden, usually semicomatose or comatose. Two nursing assistants perform this procedure together.
- ▲ Transferring a patient from a bed to a stretcher usually requires two or three nursing assistants. It is often best to do the move in several stages.
- ▲ Range-of-motion exercises are important to maintain muscle strength. The exercises move all muscles through their entire range of motion.

KNOW YOUR TERMS

MATCHING EXERCISE I

In the space provided, write the letter of the definition that best fits the numbered term.

__ 1. abduction	a. A position with the patient lying flat on the back with legs separated and knees flexed so that the soles of the feet are flat on the mattress.
__ 2. adduction	b. The straightening (of a joint).
__ 3. body alignment	c. The act of bending (usually inward).
__ 4. body mechanics	d. The moving out of or away from (said of limb moved away from the body).
__ 5. body support	e. A position with the patient lying flat on the back in bed with the legs together.
__ 6. dorsal recumbent position	f. A brace that supports the nursing assistant's back while moving patients or lifting heavy objects.
__ 7. draping	g. The moving toward (said of a limb moved toward the body).
__ 8. eversion	h. The positions, movements, and exercises that help the body maintain proper posture and avoid muscle and bone injuries.
__ 9. extension	i. A semi-sitting position with the knees slightly flexed.
__10. flexion	j. The covering of part of a patient's body with a sheet, cloth, or blanket.
__11. Fowler's position	k. A rubbing of one thing against another (as skin against bed linens).
__12. friction	l. A turning toward the inside (said of the foot).
__13. horizontal recumbent position	m. The proper positioning of the body in a line.
__14. inversion	n. Rotated outward (said of the foot).

MATCHING EXERCISE II

In the space provided, write the letter of the definition that best fits the numbered term.

__ 1. knee-chest position	a. Another name for the dorsal recumbent position.
__ 2. lateral position	b. A position with the patient lying on one side with one knee flexed slightly more than the other.
__ 3. mechanical lift	c. A position with the entire bed tilted so that the head is slightly higher than the feet.
__ 4. pronation	d. Exercises designed to move all muscles and joints through their complete range of motion.
__ 5. prone position	e. A cloth belt that buckles around a patient's waist and can be held by a nursing assistant.

___ 6. range-of-motion exercises — f. A device that raises patients in a sling from one place and transfers them to another.

___ 7. reverse Trendelenburg's position — g. A position with the patient lying face down with knees and chest touching the bed. The knees are flexed at a 90-degree angle to the bed.

___ 8. semi-Fowler's position — h. A position with the patient lying on the abdomen with the head turned to one side.

___ 9. Sim's position — i. A position with the entire bed tilted so that the feet are slightly higher than the head.

___10. stretcher — j. A position that is similar to Fowler's position, with the feet of the bed raised.

___11. supination — k. A bedlike device with wheels for transporting sick or injured people within or to the hospital.

___12. supine position — l. A turning downward (said of the wrist).

___13. transfer belt — m. A turning upward (said of the wrist).

___14. Trendelenburg's position — n. A position with the patient lying on the left side with the right knee flexed up toward the abdomen and resting on a pillow.

TEST YOUR KNOWLEDGE

Write the word(s) that best completes the statement.

1. ______________ ______________ refers to the use of the body to lift and move.
2. ______________ ______________ refers to the correct positioning of the head, back, and limbs.
3. Keep your feet ______________ inches apart when lifting heavy objects.
4. Rubbing one surface against another produces ______________.
5. ______________ is covering a patient's body with a sheet, blanket, or other material.
6. In the ______________ ______________ position, the patient is lying flat on the back with the legs close together.
7. A ______________ ______________ is put around the patient's waist for safety during transferring and walking.
8. A ______________ ______________ is used to move patients who are semicomatose or comatose.
9. ______________-______________-______________ exercises help maintain patients' muscle strength.
10. ______________ means moving away from the body.

▲ THINK ABOUT THE ISSUES

1. What are some important safety issues in transferring and moving patients?
2. Some residents or patients are bedridden and get little movement. Why are range-of-motion exercises important for such residents?

▲ CHECK YOUR SKILLS

In the following procedure checklists, check each task box that applies and answer yes or no to each step you have completed. If possible, have your instructor sign off when you have completed a procedure.

PROCEDURE

OBRA

MOVING A PATIENT UP IN BED WHO CAN ASSIST YOU

Standard Precautions ☐ Handwashing ☐ Gloving ☐ Gowning ☐ Masking

Introductory Tasks ☐ Gather Equipment ☐ Identify/Introduce/Explain ☐ Provide Privacy

	Yes	No
6. Check to make sure the wheels of the bed are locked.	___	___
7. If the bed is a hospital bed, raise it to a working height (approximately waist high) that is appropriate for good body mechanics.	___	___
8. Lower the head of the bed. If appropriate for the patient, the bed should be totally flat.	___	___
9. If the patient can be without it, move the pillow up against the headboard to protect the patient's head during the move.	___	___
10. Make sure the rail on the far side of the bed is in a raised and locked position. Lower the side rail near you.	___	___
11. Before you begin the actual move, ask for the patient's cooperation. Ask the patient to bend his or her knees and put the feet flat on the bed. The patient may also put the hand away from you flat on the bed and use it to help push off.	___	___
12. If possible, ask the patient to place the arm closest to you under your arm and behind your shoulder. The patient's hand should rest on your shoulder.	___	___
13. Place your arm under the patient's arm that is closest to you. Your hand is on the patient's shoulder.	___	___
14. Place your other arm gently under the patient's neck and shoulders.	___	___
15. On the count of three, pull the patient up to a sitting position or semi-sitting position, if appropriate. If not, the patient can be pulled to a prone position.	___	___

	Yes	No
16. Now use your free arm to do the task you need to do—tie the patient's gown, readjust the pillow, and so on.	___	___
17. After you finish the task, help the patient lie back down. With your locked arm, provide support to the patient. Use your other arm to support the neck and shoulders.	___	___
18. Check to make sure the patient is comfortable and that his or her spine is straight.	___	___
19. Place the pillow under the patient's head, straighten the bed linens, and make sure the signal light is within the patient's reach.	___	___
20. Raise the side rail on your side of the bed, if specified for the patient.	___	___
21. Lower the bed.	___	___
22. Open the screen (the curtain).	___	___
23. Wash your hands.	___	___

Procedure Completed ______________________ **Date** ______________

Notes ____

____

____

PROCEDURE

OBRA SP

MOVING A HELPLESS PATIENT IN BED

Standard Precautions ☐ Handwashing ☐ Gloving ☐ Gowning ☐ Masking

Introductory Tasks ☐ Gather Equipment ☐ Identify/Introduce/Explain ☐ Provide Privacy

	Yes	No
7. Check that the bed's wheels are locked.	___	___
8. If possible, raise the bed to a working height that is appropriate for good body mechanics.	___	___
9. Lower the head of the bed. If appropriate for the patient, the bed should be totally flat.	___	___
10. If the patient can be without it, move the pillow up against the headboard to protect the patient's head during the move.	___	___
11. Ask your helper to stand on one side of the bed. Stand on the opposite side.	___	___
12. If appropriate, lower the side rails.	___	___
13. Before you begin the actual move, ask for the patient's cooperation.	___	___

	Yes	No
14. Place your feet about 12 inches apart. Have one foot pointed toward the head of the bed and the other foot pointed toward the side of the bed. Bend your knees, and keep your back straight.	___	___
15. Place your arm under the patient's shoulder closest to you. Place your other arm under the patient's hips. Ask your helper to do the same on the other side.	___	___
16. Hold your helper's forearm and have the helper hold yours.	___	___
17. Ask the patient to bend and slightly raise both knees. Assist the patient if necessary.	___	___
18. Explain that, on the count of three, you and your helper are going to pull the patient up toward the head of the bed. If able, the patient can assist by pushing against the mattress with both feet.	___	___
19. On the count of three, move the patient up in the bed.	___	___
20. If the patient has not moved as far as necessary, repeat Steps 14 through 19.	___	___
21. Place the pillow under the patient's head.	___	___
22. Check to make sure the patient is comfortable and that his or her spine is straight.	___	___
23. Straighten the bed linens and make sure the signal light is within the patient's reach.	___	___
24. Raise the side rails, if specified for the patient.	___	___
25. Lower the bed.	___	___
26. Open the screen.	___	___
27. Wash your hands.	___	___

Procedure Completed ______________________________ **Date** ____________________

Notes ____

____

____

PROCEDURE

OBRA

MOVING A PATIENT USING A TURNING SHEET (OR DRAW SHEET)

Standard Precautions ☐ Handwashing ☐ Gloving ☐ Gowning ☐ Masking

Introductory Tasks ☐ Gather Equipment ☐ Identify/Introduce/Explain ☐ Provide Privacy

	Yes	No
7. Check to make sure the wheels of the bed are locked.	___	___
8. If possible, raise the bed to a working height that is appropriate for good body mechanics.	___	___
9. Lower the head of the bed. If appropriate for the patient, the bed should be as flat as possible.	___	___
10. If the patient can be without it, move the pillow up against the headboard to protect the patient's head during the move.	___	___
11. Ask your helper to stand on one side of the bed. Stand on the opposite side.	___	___
12. Make sure the rails are down.	___	___
13. Before you begin the actual move, ask for the patient's cooperation.	___	___
14. Roll both sides of the turning sheet up against the patient.	___	___
15. With one hand, firmly grasp the turning sheet near the patient's buttocks. Use the other hand to do the same near the patient's shoulder.	___	___
16. Place your feet about 12 inches apart, bend your knees, and keep your back straight.	___	___
17. Explain that, on the count of three, you and your helper are going to pull the patient up toward the head of the bed.	___	___
18. On the count of three, move the patient up in the bed.	___	___
19. Unroll the turning sheet.	___	___
20. Place the pillow under the patient's head.	___	___
21. Check to make sure the patient is comfortable and has a straight spine.	___	___
22. Straighten the bed linens, raise the head of the bed to a comfortable position, and make sure the signal light is within the patient's reach.	___	___
23. Raise the side rails to a locked position, if specified.	___	___
24. Lower the bed.	___	___
25. Open the screen.	___	___
26. Wash your hands.	___	___

Procedure Completed ______________________ **Date** ______________________

Notes ____

____

____

PROCEDURE

OBRA

ROLLING A PATIENT TOWARD YOU AND POSITIONING ONTO SIDE

Standard Precautions ☐ Handwashing ☐ Gloving ☐ Gowning ☐ Masking

Introductory Tasks ☐ Gather Equipment ☐ Identify/Introduce/Explain ☐ Provide Privacy

	Yes	No
6. Check to make sure the wheels of the bed are locked.	___	___
7. If possible, raise the bed to a working height that is appropriate for good body mechanics (approximately waist high).	___	___
8. Lower the head of the bed. The bed should be as flat as possible.	___	___
9. Make sure the side rail on the opposite side of the bed is raised and in a locked position. Lower the side rail near you.	___	___
10. Position your feet about 12 inches apart and flex your knees.	___	___
11. Before you begin the actual move, ask for the patient's cooperation. Explain that the move will not take place all at once, but in several steps.	___	___
12. Cross the patient's arms over the chest.	___	___
13. Position one arm under the patient's neck and shoulders.	___	___
14. Place your other arm under the middle of the patient's back.	___	___
15. Grasp the patient's far shoulder with your hand and move the patient's upper body toward you. As you do, shift your weight to your back leg.	___	___
16. Put one of your arms under the patient's thigh and the other under the patient's waist.	___	___
17. Move the patient's lower body toward you. As you do, shift your weight onto your back leg.	___	___
18. Put one of your arms under the patient's calf and the other under the patient's feet.	___	___
19. Move the patient's lower legs and feet toward you. As you do, shift your weight onto your back leg.	___	___
20. If the patient needs to be turned onto his or her side also, complete Steps 21 and 22. If the patient does not need to be turned, go to Step 23.	___	___
21. Place your hand on the patient's shoulder and hip that are on the far side of the bed.	___	___

	Yes	No
22. Gently roll the patient toward you.	___	___
23. Check to make sure the patient is comfortable and that the body is aligned properly.	___	___
24. Position pillows for the patient's comfort and support. **a.** Place a pillow under the patient's head and shoulders. **b.** Place a pillow against the patient's back. **c.** Place a pillow between the patient's legs. Gently flex the knee of the top leg. **d.** Place a small pillow under the patient's hand and arm.	___	___
25. Straighten the bed linens and make sure the signal light is within the patient's reach.	___	___
26. Raise the side rail on your side of the bed, if specified for the patient.	___	___
27. Lower the bed.	___	___
28. Open the screen.	___	___
29. Wash your hands.	___	___

Procedure Completed ______________________ **Date** ______________

Notes ____

____

____

PROCEDURE

OBRA SP

TURNING OR ROLLING A PATIENT AWAY FROM YOU AND POSITIONING ONTO SIDE

	Yes	No
1. Complete Steps 1 through 12 in Procedure, Rolling a Patient Toward You and Positioning Onto Side.	___	___
2. Put one hand under the patient's shoulder that is closest to you and the other under the patient's buttocks.	___	___
3. Gently push the patient toward the far side of the bed. As you do, shift your weight to your front leg.	___	___
4. Check to make sure the patient is comfortable and that the body is aligned properly.	___	___
5. Position pillows for the patient's comfort and support. **a.** Place a pillow under the patient's head and shoulders. **b.** Place a pillow against the patient's back. **c.** Place a pillow on the bed in front of or on top of the bottom leg. Gently flex the knee of the top leg and place the leg on the pillow. **d.** Place a small pillow under the patient's hand and arm.	___	___

	Yes	No
6. Straighten the bed linens and make sure the signal light is within the patient's reach.	___	___
7. Raise the side rail on your side of the bed.	___	___
8. Lower the bed.	___	___
9. Open the screen.	___	___
10. Wash your hands.	___	___

Procedure Completed ______________________ **Date** ______________________

Notes ____

____

____

PROCEDURE OBRA SP

LOGROLLING A PATIENT AND POSITIONING ONTO SIDE

Standard Precautions ☐ Handwashing ☐ Gloving ☐ Gowning ☐ Masking

Introductory Tasks ☐ Gather Equipment ☐ Identify/Introduce/Explain ☐ Provide Privacy

	Yes	No
7. Check to make sure the wheels of the bed are locked.	___	___
8. If possible, raise the bed to a working height that is appropriate for good body mechanics.	___	___
9. Lower the head of the bed. The bed should be as flat as possible.	___	___
10. Make sure the rail is up on the side of the bed toward which the patient will be turned. Lower the side rail near you.	___	___
11. Before you begin the actual move, ask for the patient's cooperation.	___	___
12. Using the turning sheet and with your helper's assistance, move the patient to the side of the bed near you.	___	___
13. Place a pillow or two between the patient's legs.	___	___
14. Position the patient's arms crossed on the chest.	___	___
15. Raise the rail on the side of the bed where you are working. Go to the other side of the bed and lower the side rail.	___	___
16. Stand near the patient's upper body. Ask your helper to stand by the patient's waist and thighs, on the same side of the bed.	___	___
17. Position your feet about 12 inches apart. Place one foot in front of the other.	___	___

	Yes	No
18. If the patient can assist, ask him or her to keep the body as rigid as possible during the rolling.	___	___
19. In cooperation with your helper, roll the patient toward you. You may also use a turning sheet for this procedure.	___	___
20. Check to make sure the patient is comfortable and that the body is aligned properly.	___	___
21. Position pillows for the patient's comfort and support. **a.** If appropriate for the patient's condition, place a pillow under the patient's head and shoulders. **b.** Place a pillow against the patient's back. **c.** Place a pillow on the bed over the knee of the bottom leg. Gently flex the knee of the top leg and place the leg on the pillow. **d.** Place a small pillow under the patient's hand and arm.	___	___
22. Straighten the bed linens and make sure the signal light is within the patient's reach.	___	___
23. Raise the side rail on your side of the bed.	___	___
24. Lower the bed.	___	___
25. Open the screen.	___	___
26. Wash your hands.	___	___

Procedure Completed ______________________ **Date** ______________________

Notes ____

____

____

PROCEDURE

OBRA SP

HELPING A PATIENT SIT AND DANGLE

Standard Precautions ☐ Handwashing ☐ Gloving ☐ Gowning ☐ Masking

Introductory Tasks ☐ Gather Equipment ☐ Identify/Introduce/Explain ☐ Provide Privacy

	Yes	No
6. Decide which side of the bed the patient will sit on.	___	___
7. Check to make sure the wheels of the bed are locked.	___	___
8. Raise the bed to a working height that is appropriate for good body mechanics.	___	___
9. If the patient is not positioned properly in bed, help the patient move up in bed.	___	___

	Yes	No
10. Fanfold the top linens down to the foot of the bed.	___	___
11. If the patient can move in bed, ask the patient to move to the side of the bed. Provide assistance as necessary.	___	___
12. Raise the head of the bed until the patient is sitting up.	___	___
13. Place one arm under the patient's neck and shoulders. Place your other arm under the patient's knees.	___	___
14. Gently turn the patient so the legs hang over the edge of the bed. This is "dangling."	___	___
15. Observe the patient's condition. (Check the pulse and respirations.) Help a patient who does not feel well, is breathing with difficulty, or is uncomfortable sitting up, to lie back down immediately.	___	___
16. Stay with the patient while he or she is sitting up.	___	___
17. Assist the patient in putting on a robe and slippers, if appropriate. The robe should be nearby. Never leave the patient alone.	___	___
18. When the patient is ready to lie down, reverse the steps you followed to move the patient into a sitting position.	___	___
19. Once the patient is back in the center of the bed, lower the head of the bed to an appropriate position.	___	___
20. Check to make sure the patient is comfortable and that the body is aligned properly.	___	___
21. Cover the patient with the top linens that were fanfolded to the foot of the bed.	___	___
22. Make sure the signal light is within the patient's reach.	___	___
23. Raise the side rail on the side of the bed where the patient had been sitting.	___	___
24. Lower the bed.	___	___
25. Open the screen.	___	___
26. Wash your hands.	___	___

Procedure Completed ______________________ **Date** ______________

Notes ____

____

____

PROCEDURE

OBRA SP

USING A MECHANICAL LIFT

Standard Precautions	☐ Handwashing	☐ Gloving	☐ Gowning	☐ Masking
Introductory Tasks	☐ Gather Equipment	☐ Identify/Introduce/Explain	☐ Provide Privacy	

Step	Yes	No
7. Center the sling of the mechanical lift under the patient. To get the sling under the patient, move him or her as you would if you were making an occupied bed (see Chapter 14). The lower edge of the sling should be positioned underneath the patient's knees.	___	___
8. Position the wheelchair (with locked wheels) or armchair alongside the head of the bed on the side where you will be working. Fold a bath blanket or other cover and place it in the chair. A cushion may also be used.	___	___
9. Lower the bed to its lowest position. Check to make sure the wheels of the bed are locked.	___	___
10. Raise the head of the bed to bring the patient into a sitting position.	___	___
11. Move the release valve on the lift to the closed position.	___	___
12. Raise the lift so it can be positioned over the patient.	___	___
13. Spread the legs of the lift to provide a solid base of support. The legs *must* be locked in this position, or the lift may topple over with the resident in it and hurt both the patient and the nursing assistants.	___	___
14. Move the lift into position over the patient.	___	___
15. Fasten the sling to the straps or chains. Turn the hooks away from the patient.	___	___
16. Attach the sling to the swivel bar with the short side attached to the top of the sling and the long side attached to the bottom of the sling.	___	___
17. Cross the patient's arms across the chest. The patient may hold on to the straps. (Do not let the patient hold on to the swivel bar.)	___	___
18. Raise the lift until the patient and the sling are clear of the bed.	___	___
19. Have your helper support the patient's legs as you move the lift from the bed to the chair.	___	___
20. Turn the patient so he or she is facing the mast and is centered over the base.	___	___
21. Position the lift so the patient's back is facing toward the chair.	___	___
22. Move the lift so the patient is over the seat of the chair.	___	___
23. Slowly open the release valve on the lift. Gently lower the patient into the chair.	___	___
24. Lower the bar enough so you can unhook the sling. Leave the sling under the patient.	___	___
25. Place slippers on the patient's feet. If using a wheelchair, position the patient's feet on the footrests.	___	___

	Yes	No
26. Place a covering over the patient's lap and legs if necessary.	___	___
27. Arrange the signal light so that the patient can easily reach it.	___	___
28. Wash your hands.	___	___
29. Report your observations to the nurse, including how the patient tolerated the activity, and any complaints of dizziness, difficulty breathing, weakness, and so on.	___	___
30. When the patient is ready to return to bed, reverse the procedure.	___	___

Procedure Completed ______________________ **Date** ______________________

Notes ____

____

____

PROCEDURE

OBRA SP

APPLYING A TRANSFER BELT

Standard Precautions ☐ Handwashing ☐ Gloving ☐ Gowning ☐ Masking

Introductory Tasks ☐ Gather Equipment ☐ Identify/Introduce/Explain ☐ Provide Privacy

	Yes	No
6. Help the patient move to a sitting position.	___	___
7. Place the transfer belt around the patient's waist, over the patient's clothes.	___	___
8. Position the buckle off center in the front or to the side, but never at the patient's back.	___	___
9. Tighten the belt snugly around the patient's waist. Do not make the belt too tight; it should not interfere with breathing or comfort. Two of your fingers should fit comfortably under the belt.	___	___
10. Wash your hands.	___	___

Procedure Completed ______________________ **Date** ______________________

Notes ____

____

____

PROCEDURE

OBRA SP

TRANSFERRING A PATIENT TO A WHEELCHAIR

Standard Precautions	☐ Handwashing	☐ Gloving	☐ Gowning	☐ Masking
Introductory Tasks	☐ Gather Equipment	☐ Identify/Introduce/Explain	☐ Provide Privacy	

	Yes	No
6. Decide which side of the bed you will use. If necessary, move furniture to clear enough room to work. Always put the wheelchair on the patient's strong side, if the patient is a hemiplegic or has an impairment on one side.	___	___
7. If possible, position the wheelchair alongside the head of the bed on the side where you will be working. The front of the chair should face the front of the bed with one side of the chair put firmly against the side of the bed. Use your common sense if furniture is in the way. Place the wheelchair wherever you are best able to help the patient into the chair.	___	___
8. If the patient needs it, put a cushion, soaker pad, bath blanket, sheepskin pad, or other covering on the seat of the chair. Most residents should not sit directly on the plastic seat for extended periods. Make sure the wheels are locked and the footrests are in the raised position.	___	___
9. Move the bed to its lowest position and check to make sure the wheels of the bed are locked.	___	___
10. Fanfold the top bed linens down to the foot of the bed.	___	___
11. Position the paper or sheet under the patient's feet. Put shoes or slippers on the patient's feet.	___	___
12. Help the patient move to the edge of the bed and dangle his or her feet over the edge of the bed. Be sure the patient's feet touch the floor.	___	___
13. Help the patient put on a robe.	___	___
14. If you will be using a transfer belt, apply it now.	___	___
15. Help the patient move to a standing position.	___	___

When using a transfer belt, follow steps (a) through (e):

a. Position yourself in front of the patient.
b. Have the patient put his or her hands on your shoulders, not around your neck.
c. Grab hold of both sides of the transfer belt.
d. Brace the patient by blocking the patient's knees with your knee and the patient's feet with your foot.
e. As you straighten your knees, raise the patient into a standing position.

When not using a transfer belt, follow steps (f) through (j):

f. Position yourself in front of the patient.
g. Put your hands under the patient's arms so your hands are around the patient's shoulder blades.
h. Brace the patient by blocking the patient's knees with your knee and the patient's feet with your foot.

	Yes	No
i. Ask the patient to assist you by making fists with both hands. On the count of three, ask the patient to push both fists into the mattress and lean forward.		
j. On the count of three, straighten your knees and raise the patient to a standing position.		
16. While the patient is standing, either hold the transfer belt or continue to brace the patient's knees and feet.	___	___
17. Move the patient into a position where he or she can reach the arm on the far side of the wheelchair.	___	___
18. Slowly turn the patient so he or she can reach and hold the other arm of the wheelchair.	___	___
19. Ask the patient to cooperate by flexing the knees and elbows and leaning forward. Have the patient touch the front of the wheelchair seat with the back of the knees before sitting. Gently lower the patient into the wheelchair. As you do, be sure to flex your knees and hips.	___	___
20. Position the patient comfortably and in good body alignment. The patient's buttocks should be positioned far back on the seat.	___	___
21. Arrange the patient's feet on the wheelchair footrests.	___	___
22. You may place a bath blanket over the patient's lap and legs if necessary. Check to make sure the blanket is not hanging on the floor or over the wheels of the wheelchair. Make sure the patient is secured in the wheelchair (if necessary).	___	___
23. If you used a transfer belt, remove it.	___	___
24. Arrange the signal light so the patient can easily reach it.	___	___
25. Wash your hands.	___	___
26. Report your observations to the nurse, including how the patient tolerated the activity, the pulse (if taken), and any complaints of dizziness, difficulty breathing, weakness, and so on.	___	___
27. When the patient is ready to return to bed, reverse the procedure.	___	___

Procedure Completed ______________________ **Date** ______________________

Notes ____

____

____

PROCEDURE

OBRA SP

TRANSFERRING A PATIENT TO A WHEELCHAIR WITH A HELPER

Standard Precautions	☐ Handwashing	☐ Gloving	☐ Gowning	☐ Masking
Introductory Tasks	☐ Gather Equipment	☐ Identify/Introduce/Explain	☐ Provide Privacy	

Step	Yes	No
6. Decide which side of the bed you will use. If necessary, move small items of furniture to clear enough room to work.	___	___
7. Position the wheelchair alongside the head of the bed on the side where you will be working. The front of the chair should face the front of the bed.	___	___
8. Fold a bath blanket and place it in the chair. Make sure the wheels are locked and the footrests are in the raised position.	___	___
9. Move the bed to its lowest position and check to make sure the wheels of the bed are locked.	___	___
10. Fanfold the top bed linens down to the foot of the bed.	___	___
11. Help the patient move to the side of the bed near the wheelchair. Raise the head of the bed so the patient is in a sitting position.	___	___
12. Position yourself in front of the wheelchair at the head of the bed.	___	___
13. Put your arms around the patient's waist.	___	___
14. Ask your helper to place his or her arms under the patient's legs.	___	___
15. On the count of three, move the patient toward the wheelchair and gently lower him or her into the wheelchair.	___	___
16. Position the patient comfortably and in good body alignment. The patient's buttocks should be positioned far back on the seat.	___	___
17. Arrange the patient's feet on the wheelchair footrests.	___	___
18. You may place a bath blanket over the patient's lap and legs if necessary. Check to make sure the blanket is not hanging on the floor or over the wheels of the wheelchair. Make sure the patient is secured in the wheelchair, according to facility policy.	___	___
19. Arrange the signal light so the patient can easily reach it.	___	___
20. Wash your hands.	___	___
21. Report your observations to the nurse, including how the patient tolerated the activity, the pulse (if taken), and any complaints of dizziness, difficulty breathing, weakness, and so on.	___	___
22. When the patient is ready to return to bed, reverse the procedure.	___	___

Procedure Completed ______________________ **Date** ______________

Notes ____

____

____

PROCEDURE

TRANSFERRING A CONSCIOUS PATIENT TO A STRETCHER

Standard Precautions ☐ Handwashing ☐ Gloving ☐ Gowning ☐ Masking

Introductory Tasks ☐ Gather Equipment ☐ Identify/Introduce/Explain ☐ Provide Privacy

Step	Yes	No
7. Decide which side of the bed you will use.	___	___
8. If necessary, move furniture to clear enough room to work.	___	___
9. Raise the bed to a height even with the stretcher and lock the bed wheels.	___	___
10. Fanfold the top linens down to the foot of the bed.	___	___
11. Place a bath blanket over the patient's body up to the shoulders.	___	___
12. Lower the side rail on the side of the bed where the stretcher will be positioned.	___	___
13. Position the stretcher parallel to the bed, up against the bed.	___	___
14. Lock the wheels of the stretcher.	___	___
15. Ask one of your helpers to go to the opposite side of the bed and lower the side rail. Ask the other helper to stand on the far side of the stretcher to prevent it from moving.	___	___
16. Go behind the headboard of the bed and place your hands gently under the patient's pillow.	___	___
17. Ask your helper who is alongside the bed to gently place his or her hands under the patient's back and lower legs. The helper on the far side of the stretcher should place his or her hands under the patient's back and legs also.	___	___
18. The patient may be turned or moved closer to the stretcher as one move, and then, on the count of three, help the patient move onto the stretcher.	___	___
19. Fasten the stretcher straps and raise both side rails on the stretcher.	___	___
20. Wash your hands.	___	___

Procedure Completed ______________________ **Date** ______________

Notes ____

____

____

PROCEDURE

TRANSFERRING AN UNCONSCIOUS PATIENT TO A STRETCHER

Standard Precautions ☐ Handwashing ☐ Gloving ☐ Gowning ☐ Masking

Introductory Tasks ☐ Gather Equipment ☐ Identify/Introduce/Explain ☐ Provide Privacy

	Yes	No
7. Decide which side of the bed you will use. If necessary, move furniture to clear enough room to work.	___	___
8. Raise the bed to a height even with the stretcher.	___	___
9. Fanfold the top linens down to the foot of the bed.	___	___
10. Place a bath blanket over the patient's body up to the shoulders.	___	___
11. Position yourself and your helpers as follows: **a.** One helper on the far side of the bed. **b.** One against the far side of the stretcher. **c.** One at the head of the stretcher facing toward the foot of the stretcher. **d.** The nursing assistant at the foot of the bed, facing the head of the bed.	___	___
12. Lower the side rails on both sides of the bed.	___	___
13. Position the stretcher parallel to the bed, up against the bed.	___	___
14. Lock the wheels of the stretcher. Make sure the wheels of the bed are locked also.	___	___
15. Roll in both sides of the turning sheet close to the patient's body.	___	___
16. On the count of three, have all helpers carry out the following procedures at the same time: **a.** The helper at the foot of the bed raises the patient's lower legs and feet. **b.** The helper against the far side of the bed grasps and raises the turning sheet. **c.** The helper on the far side of the stretcher grasps the turning sheet with both hands, raises the sheet, and guides the patient toward the stretcher. **d.** The helper at the head of the stretcher positions both arms together under the patient's shoulders to support the patient's head and neck.	___	___
17. Position the patient in the center of the stretcher.	___	___
18. Fasten the stretcher restraints.	___	___
19. Raise and lock the side rails on the stretcher.	___	___
20. Wash your hands.	___	___

Procedure Completed ______________________ **Date** ______________

Notes ____

____

____

PROCEDURE

OBRA SP

PERFORMING RANGE-OF-MOTION EXERCISES

Standard Precautions ☐ Handwashing ☐ Gloving ☐ Gowning ☐ Masking

Introductory Tasks ☐ Gather Equipment ☐ Identify/Introduce/Explain ☐ Provide Privacy

	Yes	No
6. Raise the bed to a position that allows for good body mechanics.	___	___
7. Lower both side rails.	___	___
8. Place the patient in a supine position.	___	___
9. Fanfold top linens down to the foot of the bed.	___	___
10. Cover the patient with a bath blanket.	___	___
11. Exercise the patient's toes: **a.** Curl the toes (flexion). **b.** Straighten the toes (extension). **c.** Spread the toes apart (abduction). **d.** Pull the toes together (adduction). **e.** Repeat steps (a) through (d) the number of times indicated by your supervisor.	___	___
12. Exercise the patient's foot: **a.** Turn the inside of the foot down and the outside of the foot up (eversion). **b.** Turn the inside of the foot up and the outside of the foot down (inversion). **c.** Repeat steps (a) and (b) the number of times indicated by your supervisor.	___	___
13. Exercise the patient's ankle: **a.** Position one hand under the patient's foot and the other under the ankle. **b.** At the same time, pull the foot forward and push the heel down (dorsiflexion). **c.** Point the toes forward or turn the foot down (plantar flexion). **d.** Repeat steps (a) through (c) the number of times indicated by your supervisor.	___	___
14. Exercise the patient's knee: **a.** Position one hand under the patient's knee and the other under the ankle. **b.** Bend the leg (flexion). **c.** Straighten the leg (extension). **d.** Repeat steps (a) through (c) the number of times indicated by your supervisor.	___	___
15. Exercise the patient's hip: **a.** Position one hand under the patient's knee and the other under the ankle. **b.** Raise the leg (flexion).	___	___

	Yes	No
c. Straighten the leg (extension). **d.** Move the leg away from the body (abduction). **e.** Move the leg toward the body (adduction). **f.** Turn the leg inward (internal rotation). **g.** Turn the leg outward (external rotation). **h.** Repeat steps (a) through (g) the number of times indicated by your supervisor.		
16. Exercise the fingers: **a.** Spread the fingers and thumb apart (abduction). **b.** Move the fingers and thumb together (adduction). **c.** Straighten the fingers out (extension). **d.** Make a fist (flexion). **e.** Repeat steps (a) through (d) the number of times indicated by your supervisor.	___	___
17. Exercise the thumb: **a.** With one hand, hold the patient's hand. With your other hand, hold the patient's thumb. **b.** Move the thumb away from the index finger (abduction). **c.** Move the thumb toward the index finger (adduction). **d.** Bend the thumb in toward the palm of the hand (flexion). **e.** Move the thumb out to the side of the fingers (extension). **f.** Move the thumb to touch the tip of each finger (opposition). **g.** Repeat steps (a) through (f) the number of times indicated by your supervisor.	___	___
18. Exercise the patient's wrist: **a.** Hold the patient's wrist with both of your hands. **b.** Move one of your hands forward and bend the patient's hand downward (flexion). **c.** Straighten out the hand (extension). **d.** Bend the hand back (hyperextension). **e.** Turn the wrist and hand toward the thumb (radial flexion). **f.** Turn the wrist and hand toward the pinky finger (ulnar flexion). **g.** Repeat steps (a) through (f) the number of times indicated by your supervisor.	___	___
19. Exercise the patient's forearm: **a.** Turn the patient's hand so the palm faces down (pronation). **b.** Turn the hand so the palm faces up (supination). **c.** Repeat steps (a) and (b) the number of times indicated by your supervisor.	___	___
20. Exercise the patient's elbow: **a.** Hold the patient's wrist with one hand. Hold the patient's elbow with your other hand. **b.** Bend the patient's arm so it touches the shoulder on the same side of the body (flexion). **c.** Straighten the arm (extension). **d.** Repeat steps (a) through (c) the number of times indicated by your supervisor.	___	___
21. Exercise the patient's shoulder: **a.** Hold the patient's wrist with one hand. Hold the patient's elbow with your other hand. **b.** Raise the patient's arm out straight in front of the body and up over the head (abduction). **c.** Lower the arm down to the patient's side (adduction). **d.** If the patient is standing or sitting in a chair, move the patient's arm behind the body (hyperextension).	___	___

	Yes	No
e. Move the patient's straight arm up and away from the side of the body (abduction). **f.** Move the straight arm down to the side of the body (adduction). **g.** Bend the patient's elbow and position it at shoulder height. Move the forearm down and toward the body (internal rotation). **h.** Move the forearm toward the head (external rotation). **i.** Repeat steps (a) through (h) the number of times indicated by your supervisor.		
22. Exercise the patient's neck: **a.** Position your hands on the patient's head as shown. **b.** Move the patient's head forward until the chin touches the chest (flexion). **c.** Straighten the head (extension). **d.** Move the head backward so that the chin points upward (hyperextension). **e.** Turn the head to one side and then to the other side (rotation). **f.** Move the head to the right and then to the left (lateral flexion). **g.** Repeat steps (a) through (f) the number of times indicated by your supervisor.	___	___
23. Go to the other side of the bed or chair and repeat Steps 11 through 22 for the limbs and joints on the other side of the patient's body.	___	___
24. Check to make sure the patient is comfortable and that the body is aligned properly.	___	___
25. Unfold the top linens and cover the patient. Straighten the bed linens.	___	___
26. Remove the bath blanket.	___	___
27. Make sure the signal light is within the patient's reach.	___	___
28. Raise the side rails of the bed.	___	___
29. Lower the bed.	___	___
30. Open the screen.	___	___
31. Wash your hands.	___	___
32. Report and record the following information: • The time of the exercises • The joints exercised and the number of times • Any complaints of pain • The degree to which the patient participated	___	___

Procedure Completed ______________________ **Date** ______________

Notes ____

____

____

CHAPTER 17

PATIENT REHABILITATION

STUDY OBJECTIVES

Rehabilitation is the process of restoring patients to the highest possible level of functioning and ability. The nursing assistant plays a role in helping patients participate fully in rehabilitation.

- The nursing assistant's role in rehabilitation is to support and encourage the patient, provide care, and help in performing any rehabilitation activities that are assigned by a doctor, therapist, or nurse.
- The nursing assistant provides personal care for a patient in traction. Observing the patient while giving care is a valuable part of the care process. Patients in traction often require help in positioning themselves.
- Casts, braces, and splints immobilize and support injured or disabled body parts to allow healing or to prevent further damage. Cast and splint care includes observation for abnormalities and keeping the patient as comfortable as possible.
- Walking aids help patients achieve some degree of mobility. They provide a measure of safety for patients with some weakness of the legs. Avoiding falls is an important responsibility of everyone on the health care team. Some falls are not preventable, and nursing assistants need to know how to support a falling patient.
- Different types of walking aids include canes, walkers, braces, and crutches.

KNOW YOUR TERMS

In the space provided, write the letter of the definition that best fits the numbered term.

__ 1. brace	a. The process of restoring someone to his or her prior or best capacity after an injury or illness.
__ 2. cane	b. A walking aid, usually used in pairs, that fits under the arm.
__ 3. cast	c. A break in a bone.
__ 4. crutch	d. A sticklike device used for support while walking.
__ 5. fracture	e. A program of exercise and nutrition meant to restore someone to his or her best capacity.
__ 6. rehabilitation program	f. A device, usually fitted to a limb, used as a walking aid.
__ 7. restorative care	g. A device made of plaster, plastic, or fiberglass that immobilizes a part of the body during healing.
__ 8. splint	h. A device with four legs and a top rail, used as a walking aid.
__ 9. traction	i. A device, often made of cloth, used to immobilize a body part for a short time.
__10. walker	j. Any device that aids a patient in walking.
__11. walking aid	k. The exertion of a pulling force to maintain proper bone alignment.

TEST YOUR KNOWLEDGE

Write the word(s) that best completes each statement.

1. A physical therapist helps to set up and manage a patient's ____________ program.
2. Nursing assistants should practice measures that prevent skin ____________.
3. A rehabilitation program usually involves ____________ of specific exercises.
4. Traction is used to treat ____________.
5. Traction can be applied ____________ or ____________.
6. Skin ____________ may develop around and under casts.
7. Warm skin around a cast may signal an ____________.
8. Cold skin around a cast may signal a ____________ problem.
9. Patients should not ____________ any items in their hands while using a walker.
10. You may not be able to ____________ falls due to patient dizziness, fainting, or weakness.

▲ THINK ABOUT THE ISSUES

1. There is a fine line between encouraging a patient in rehabilitation to do more and pushing a patient too fast. Always follow the instructions of the other members of the health care team. Sometimes, those instructions may seem to push a patient too fast or hold a patient back who is anxious to proceed. How should a nursing assistant handle situations that seem too fast or too slow for the patient?
2. A patient with a chronic, debilitating disease wishes to continue walking with a walking aid rather than accepting the need for a wheelchair. Should you encourage the patient to walk, or should you offer the wheelchair at frequent intervals?

▲ CHECK YOUR SKILLS

In the following procedure checklists, check each task box that applies and answer yes or no to each step you have completed. If possible, have your instructor sign off when you have completed a procedure.

PROCEDURE

OBRA SP

USING A TRANSFER BELT TO HELP A PATIENT WALK

Standard Precautions ☐ Handwashing ☐ Gloving ☐ Gowning ☐ Masking

Introductory Tasks ☐ Gather Equipment ☐ Identify/Introduce/Explain ☐ Provide Privacy

	Yes	No
6. Make sure there is adequate lighting and a pathway free of objects.	___	___
7. Decide which side of the bed to use. Get the patient out of bed on the strong side, if possible.	___	___
8. Check to make sure the wheels of the bed are locked.	___	___
9. If the bed can be raised or lowered, lower the bed to a working height that is comfortable for you, and low enough for the patient to get up easily.	___	___
10. If necessary, help the patient move up in bed to a proper position.	___	___
11. Fanfold the top linens down to the foot of the bed.	___	___
12. If possible, position the sheet or paper under the patient's feet on the bed.	___	___
13. Place the patient's nonskid slippers or shoes on both feet.	___	___
14. If the patient can move in bed, ask him or her to move to the side of the bed. Provide assistance if necessary.	___	___
15. Raise the side rail on the side of the bed that is furthest from the patient.	___	___
16. Raise the head of the bed until the patient is sitting up.	___	___

	Yes	No
17. If necessary, lower the rail on the side of the bed closest to the patient.	___	___
18. Help the patient to sit up in bed and dangle the feet over the edge of the bed. **a.** Slide one arm under the patient's neck and shoulders and grasp the far shoulder. Place your other hand under the far knee. **b.** Turn the patient a quarter turn. As the legs go over the edge of the mattress, the patient will be upright. **c.** Ask the patient to push both fists into the mattress as a support in the sitting position. **d.** Ask how the patient feels (that is, dizzy or lightheaded). **e.** Check the pulse and respirations. **f.** If necessary, help the patient lie back down. (Reverse the procedure to lay the patient back down.)	___	___
19. Help the patient put on a bathrobe.	___	___
20. Position the transfer belt on the patient.	___	___
21. Help the patient move to a standing position: **a.** Position yourself in front of the patient. **b.** The patient may put his or her hands flat on the bed and push off, or have the patient put his or her hands on your shoulders. Do not allow the patient to place hands around your neck—you could injure yourself or the patient. **c.** Grab hold of both sides of the transfer belt. **d.** To brace the patient, block the patient's knees with your knees and feet with your feet. **e.** On the count of three, straighten your knees and raise the patient to a standing position.	___	___
22. While the patient is standing, hold the transfer belt at the side and the back. Stand slightly behind so you can help if the patient starts to fall. Do not leave the patient alone.	___	___
23. Ask the patient to stand in a position that represents good body posture, with the head held up and the back straight.	___	___
24. When the patient is ready, help him or her to walk. Stay alongside the patient and provide support by holding onto the transfer belt. Coordinate your stride with the patient's (for example, as the patient steps forward with the left foot, step forward with your left foot).	___	___
25. Observe the patient's walking. If the patient does not appear to be walking properly (that is, shuffling the feet instead of picking them up), suggest the patient walk normally, or that he or she lift the feet.	___	___
26. Encourage the patient to walk the distance indicated by your charge nurse, therapist, or supervisor. Do not rush the patient. If the patient cannot complete the entire distance, do not force it.	___	___
27. When the walk is finished, assist the patient with returning to bed: **a.** Ask the patient to stand against the side of the bed. **b.** Turn the patient's body a quarter turn so that the back of both knees are touching the bed. **c.** Ask the patient to place both hands on the mattress or on your shoulders. (Not around your neck.) **d.** Hold onto both sides of the transfer belt.	___	___

	Yes	No
e. Gently lower the patient onto the bed, bending your knees as you do so. **f.** Remove the transfer belt. **g.** Remove the patient's bathrobe and slippers/shoes. **h.** Help the patient lie down in bed.		
28. Lower the head of the bed to a comfortable position for the patient.	___	___
29. Move the patient to the center of the bed.	___	___
30. Remove the paper or sheet under the patient's feet.	___	___
31. Check to make sure the patient is comfortable and that body alignment is correct.	___	___
32. Straighten the bed linens and make sure the signal light is within the patient's reach.	___	___
33. Raise the side rail on the side of the bed closest to you.	___	___
34. Unscreen the patient.	___	___
35. Wash your hands.	___	___
36. Report and record the following: the distance walked, and how the patient tolerated the procedure.	___	___

Procedure Completed ________________________ **Date** ____________________

Notes ____

____

____

PROCEDURE

OBRA

HELPING A PATIENT WHO IS FALLING

	Yes	No
1. Position your body in a way that offers a firm base of support. Move your feet a comfortable distance apart and straighten your back.	___	___
2. If the patient is wearing a transfer belt, grasp the belt. If there is no belt, put your arms around the patient's waist or under the arms. Pull the patient's body toward your body.	___	___
3. Position one of your legs as a rest for the patient's buttocks. Let the patient's buttocks rest on your knee.	___	___
4. Gently lower the patient to the floor by letting him or her slide down your leg. As you lower the patient, bend your knees and hips.	___	___
5. Have a charge nurse come and check the patient's condition.	___	___
6. Transport the patient back to bed. Ask several helpers to assist you if necessary.	___	___

	Yes	No
7. Put the signal light within easy reach of the patient.	___	___
8. Wash your hands.	___	___
9. Make a report of the incident, including the following in your report: **a.** The date and time of the incident **b.** An objective account of the fall **c.** The patient's reaction to the incident	___	___

Procedure Completed ______________________ **Date** ______________________

Notes ____

____

____

CHAPTER 18

PERSONAL CARE IN A LONG-TERM CARE FACILITY

STUDY OBJECTIVES

Personal care in a long-term care facility differs for ambulatory and dependent residents. Ambulatory residents usually need only light assistance and reminders. Dependent residents need partial or total care, including all personal hygiene and dressing and undressing. Personal care includes providing good skin care, hair care, dental care, all bathing and dressing, nail and foot care, and care of eyes, eyeglasses, and hearing aids.

- An ambulatory resident's normal daily hygiene includes washing hands and face, brushing teeth, using the bathroom, bathing, shaving, dressing, and undressing. Nursing assistants assist in making sure that each task is performed as necessary and in helping where needed.
- A dependent resident usually needs help to go to the toilet or to use a bedpan or urinal first thing in the morning, followed by hand and face washing. During the day, residents must be dressed and undressed, washed, have their teeth and hair brushed, and be bathed and shaved as necessary. Rooms must be cleaned and straightened.
- Oral hygiene must be performed at least twice a day for cleanliness, avoiding mouth odor, keeping the mouth moist, and leaving a pleasant taste in the mouth. Residents either brush their teeth or clean their dentures with nursing assistants helping or performing tasks as necessary.
- Hair is shampooed at least once a week. It is brushed every day.
- Bathing and showering for ambulatory residents usually require only help from the nursing assistant. Bed baths are given to patients who are bedridden.
- Male residents can shave their own faces if they are able. If not, nursing assistants shave carefully as often as necessary.
- A resident who is able to dress and undress may need little help. A resident who is dependent needs to have the gown changed by the nursing assistant. Patients with IV tubes must have the gown put on without disconnecting anything.
- Residents should dress and undress themselves, if possible. Nursing assistants may help in getting clothes and encouraging residents to dress in a neat manner. Dependent residents need to be dressed and undressed every day. If clothes get soiled, they should be changed as soon as possible.

- ▲ Male and female perineal care is the cleaning of the genital and rectal areas. Nursing assistants always wear gloves and follow procedures and facility guidelines.
- ▲ Skin should be kept dry and lotions applied as instructed by the nurse. Massaging with lotion helps avoid skin breakdown.
- ▲ Nails and feet should be kept clean and trimmed. Foot care, especially for diabetics, should be done by or under the supervision of a podiatrist.
- ▲ A back massage is given gently and in a pattern that promotes circulation, relaxation, and good skin care.
- ▲ Eyeglasses should be cleaned and returned to the resident. Artificial eyes also need to be cleaned and returned to the resident.
- ▲ Hearing aids should be removed when the resident is being bathed or washed. They must be kept clean and dry.

▲ KNOW YOUR TERMS

In the space provided, write the letter of the definition that best fits the numbered term.

__ 1. bedsore	a. An artificial replacement for teeth.
__ 2. decubitus ulcer	b. The process of making one's appearance neat.
__ 3. dentures	c. The practices that clean and maintain the mouth, teeth, and dentures.
__ 4. grooming	d. The cleanliness practices that keep someone healthy.
__ 5. hygiene	e. The area of the body between the thighs encompassing the genital and rectal areas.
__ 6. oral hygiene	f. An informal name for pressure sore.
__ 7. perineal care	g. Chronic lesion or wound that appears near a bony prominence of a patient who is not generally ambulatory. Also called decubitus ulcer, bedsore.
__ 8. perineum	h. A formal name for pressure sore, used most often by doctors and nurses.
__ 9. pressure sore	i. Cleaning and care of the perineum.

▲ TEST YOUR KNOWLEDGE

Write the word(s) that best completes the statement.

1. ____________ is the practice of cleanliness to promote good health.
2. ____________ ____________ is performed to keep the resident's teeth and mouth clean.
3. A prepackaged tooth swab with dentifrice is called a ____________.
4. ____________ helps remove plaque and tartar from the teeth.
5. Water temperature for a bath should be between ____________° F and ____________° F.

6. A _____________ bath is a special bathtub used to stimulate the muscles and skin of residents.
7. When cleaning the female perineal area, always wipe from _____________ to _____________.
8. When cleaning the male perineal area, always wipe from _____________ to _____________.
9. A _____________ _____________ is a breakdown of the skin in a specific area.
10. A hearing aid amplifies and directs _____________ into the ear.

THINK ABOUT THE ISSUES

1. Independence in personal hygiene helps to maintain a person's dignity. How can you encourage independence in residents of a nursing home?
2. Cleanliness is both a health and a self-esteem issue for residents. If you find yourself working with a resident who is resistant to being cleaned, what should you do?

CHECK YOUR SKILLS

In the following procedure checklists, check each task box that applies and answer yes or no to each step you have completed. If possible, have your instructor sign off when you have completed a procedure.

PROCEDURE

OBRA SP

HELPING AMBULATORY RESIDENTS BRUSH THEIR TEETH

Standard Precautions ☐ Handwashing ☐ Gloving ☐ Gowning ☐ Masking

Introductory Tasks ☐ Gather Equipment ☐ Identify/Introduce/Explain ☐ Provide Privacy

Step	Yes	No
6. Help the resident to the sink. If necessary, provide a chair for the resident to lean on.	___	___
7. Help the resident wash his or her hands.	___	___
8. Help the resident moisten the toothbrush and apply toothpaste. Let the resident brush his or her teeth.	___	___
9. Fill the glass with water. Instruct the resident to rinse the mouth and expectorate the water in the sink.	___	___
10. If requested, pour a small amount of mouthwash in a clean cup. Some mouthwashes need to be diluted with water. Follow the directions on the package. Give it to the resident.	___	___

	Yes	No
11. Instruct the resident to swish the mouthwash around the mouth and expectorate into the sink.	___	___
12. Give the resident a towel to dry the mouth area.	___	___
13. Assist the resident back to bed or to a chair. Make the resident comfortable and provide for safety.	___	___
14. Return to the sink. Clean the supplies and store them for the next use.	___	___
15. Unscreen the resident.	___	___
16. Wash your hands.	___	___
17. Report any unusual observations to the supervisor.	___	___

Procedure Completed ______________________ **Date** ______________________

Notes ____

____

____

PROCEDURE

OBRA SP

BRUSHING THE TEETH OF A RESIDENT ON BED REST

Standard Precautions ☐ Handwashing ☐ Gloving ☐ Gowning ☐ Masking

Introductory Tasks ☐ Gather Equipment ☐ Identify/Introduce/Explain ☐ Provide Privacy

	Yes	No
5. Position the over-bed table at a comfortable working height. Place the paper towels on top of the table. Arrange your equipment on the table.	___	___
6. Raise the head of the bed to a comfortable, upright position for the resident.	___	___
7. Place a towel across the resident's chest to protect the gown and bed linens.	___	___
8. Moisten the toothbrush and help the resident put toothpaste on it.	___	___
9. Move the over-bed table so the resident can brush easily.	___	___
10. Assist the resident in brushing the teeth and massaging the gums. First clean the upper teeth, then the lower teeth.	___	___
11. Help the resident rinse the mouth and expectorate into the emesis basin when needed.	___	___
12. When the resident is finished brushing, offer the cool tap water. Instruct the resident to rinse and to expectorate the water in the emesis basin.	___	___

	Yes	No
13. If the resident requests mouthwash, pour a small amount of mouthwash in a clean cup. The resident swishes the mouthwash and expectorates it into the emesis basin.	___	___
14. Wipe the resident's mouth.	___	___
15. Make the resident comfortable and provide for safety.	___	___
16. Clean the equipment and put it away. Wipe off the table and return it to its original position.	___	___
17. Unscreen the resident.	___	___
18. Wash your hands.	___	___
19. Report any unusual observations to the supervisor.	___	___

Procedure Completed ______________________ **Date** ______________

Notes ____

____

____

PROCEDURE

OBRA SP

BRUSHING A DEPENDENT RESIDENT'S TEETH

Standard Precautions ☐ Handwashing ☐ Gloving ☐ Gowning ☐ Masking

Introductory Tasks ☐ Gather Equipment ☐ Identify/Introduce/Explain ☐ Provide Privacy

	Yes	No
5. Position the over-bed table at a comfortable working height. Place the paper towels on top of the table. Arrange your equipment on the table.	___	___
6. Raise the head of the bed to a comfortable upright position for the resident, if possible.	___	___
7. Cover the resident's pillow with a towel. Turn the resident's head to the side, facing you, to help avoid choking and aspiration. Place a towel over the chest to protect clothing.	___	___
8. Moisten the toothbrush or toothette with water and dip in cleaning solution (mouthwash, toothpaste, or other cleaning agent). If the resident is unconscious, you will need to open the mouth. Suction toothbrushes are sometimes used to prevent aspiration of food and fluid.	___	___
9. Clean the gums, teeth, tongue, and the inside of the mouth gently and thoroughly. Rinse the toothbrush or toothette as needed.	___	___
10. Use water on a toothette to rinse the mouth.	___	___

	Yes	No
11. Dry the resident's mouth with a towel.	___	___
12. Lubricate the lips with glycerin or petroleum jelly. Use a water-soluble lubricant, according to facility policy, when oxygen is in use.	___	___
13. Make the resident comfortable and provide for safety.	___	___
14. Clean the equipment and put it away. Wipe off the table and return it to its original position.	___	___
15. Remove your gloves.	___	___
16. Unscreen the resident.	___	___
17. Wash your hands.	___	___
18. Report any unusual observations to the supervisor.	___	___

Procedure Completed ______________________ **Date** ______________________

Notes ____

____

____

PROCEDURE

OBRA SP

FLOSSING TEETH

Standard Precautions ☐ Handwashing ☐ Gloving ☐ Gowning ☐ Masking

Introductory Tasks ☐ Gather Equipment ☐ Identify/Introduce/Explain ☐ Provide Privacy

	Yes	No
5. Position the over-bed table at a comfortable working height. Place the paper towels on top of the table. Arrange your equipment on the table.	___	___
6. Raise the head of the bed to a comfortable, upright position for the resident.	___	___
7. Place a towel across the resident's chest to protect the gown and bed linens.	___	___
8. Put on gloves.	___	___
9. Break off an 18-inch piece of dental floss. Hold the dental floss between your thumb and index finger on each hand. Stretch it tight.	___	___
10. Move the floss up and down between the teeth. Change the position of the floss for each tooth. Do not force the dental floss below the gum line.	___	___
11. Offer the resident the water periodically to swish in the mouth to loosen debris. Hold the emesis basin under the resident's chin so the resident can spit out the water.	___	___
12. Wipe the resident's mouth with a towel.	___	___

	Yes	No
13. Make the resident comfortable. Provide for the resident's safety.	___	___
14. Clean the equipment and put it away. Wipe off the table and return it to its original position.	___	___
	___	___
15. Remove your gloves.	___	___
16. Unscreen the resident.	___	___
17. Wash your hands.	___	___
18. Report any unusual observations to the supervisor.	___	___

Procedure Completed ______________________ **Date** ______________________

Notes ____

____

____

PROCEDURE

OBRA SP

CARING FOR DENTURES

Standard Precautions ☐ Handwashing ☐ Gloving ☐ Gowning ☐ Masking

Introductory Tasks ☐ Gather Equipment ☐ Identify/Introduce/Explain ☐ Provide Privacy

	Yes	No
5. Ask the resident to remove the dentures and place them in the emesis basin or denture cup. If the resident is unable to remove the dentures, you will need to remove them. Put on gloves and gather the gauze squares. Grasp the upper dentures and pull slightly downward to break the suction. Gently remove the denture once the seal is broken. Place it in the emesis basin. Remove the bottom denture by grasping it and pulling slightly upward. Place it in the emesis basin.	___	___
6. Make the resident comfortable. Provide for safety. Explain that you will be right back.	___	___
7. Take the emesis basin, denture cup, denture brush, and cleaner to the sink.	___	___
8. Line the bottom of the sink with paper towels and place the emesis basin in the sink, or fill the sink with water to cushion a falling denture.	___	___
9. Place one of the dentures in the palm of your hand and rinse in cold water. If you prefer, you can grasp the denture securely between your thumb and two fingers. Brush with cleanser until all surfaces are clean. Brush dentures up and down, holding them securely to avoid dropping them. Repeat for the other denture. Dentures may also be soaked in a denture cleaning solution.	___	___

	Yes	No
10. Rinse the dentures in cool water and return them to the denture cup. Rinse the emesis basin. Take the denture cup to the resident's bedside.	___	___
11. At this time, you can help the resident brush the gums with a soft toothbrush and offer mouthwash to refresh the mouth.	___	___
12. Offer the resident the dentures. If the resident does not want the dentures, leave them in the denture cup. Fill the cup with cool water and store it in a safe place. If the resident wants the dentures, supervise or assist the resident in replacing them in the mouth.	___	___
13. To insert dentures, grasp the upper dentures with one hand. Raise the upper lip with the other hand and insert the denture. Gently press on the denture to make sure it is securely in place. Grasp the lower denture with one hand. Lower the bottom lip with the other hand and insert the denture. Gently press on the denture to make sure it is securely in place.	___	___
14. Remove gloves.	___	___
15. Make the resident comfortable and provide for the resident's safety.	___	___
16. Clean and store the equipment for the next use.	___	___
17. Unscreen the resident.	___	___
18. Wash your hands.	___	___
19. Report any unusual observations to the supervisor.	___	___

Procedure Completed ______________________ **Date** ______________________

Notes ____

____

____

PROCEDURE

OBRA SP

SHAMPOOING A BEDRIDDEN RESIDENT'S HAIR

Standard Precautions ☐ Handwashing ☐ Gloving ☐ Gowning ☐ Masking

Introductory Tasks ☐ Gather Equipment ☐ Identify/Introduce/Explain ☐ Provide Privacy

	Yes	No
5. Position the over-bed tray so it is at a comfortable working height. Assemble your equipment.	___	___
6. Raise the bed to a comfortable working height.	___	___

	Yes	No
7. Remove the pillow and place the waterproof bed protector under the resident's head. Place a towel over the resident's chest to protect the gown and bed linens.	___	___
8. Place the trough under the resident's head. One end of the trough has a hose to drain the water. Position the basin or pail on a chair under the trough to catch the water.	___	___
9. Loosen the resident's gown and fold it over at the neck.	___	___
10. Comb the hair to loosen oils.	___	___
11. Run the water until it is warm.	___	___
12. Wet the hair thoroughly. Apply a small amount of shampoo. You can cover the resident's eyes with a washcloth to protect them.	___	___
13. Work up a lather using both hands. Work from the hairline to the back of the scalp.	___	___
14. Use your fingertips to gently massage the scalp.	___	___
15. Rinse the head with warm water. Apply more shampoo and repeat if requested or needed.	___	___
16. Apply a small amount of conditioner if the resident requests it. Massage conditioner through the hair.	___	___
17. Rinse the hair thoroughly with water.	___	___
18. Gently pat dry the resident's face and forehead with a towel.	___	___
19. Wrap the hair with a large towel. Remove the trough. Remove all other equipment from the bed.	___	___
20. Change the resident's gown if necessary.	___	___
21. Comb the hair.	___	___
22. Use a hair dryer on a low setting to dry the hair. Style the hair according to the resident's request. Hold up the mirror so the resident can see the results.	___	___
23. Make the resident comfortable and provide for safety.	___	___
24. Clean and store the equipment for the next use. Discard disposable equipment.	___	___
25. Unscreen the resident.	___	___
26. Wash your hands.	___	___
27. Report any unusual observations to the supervisor.	___	___

Procedure Completed ______________________ **Date** ______________________

Notes ____

____

____

PROCEDURE

OBRA SP

HELPING AMBULATORY PATIENTS SHOWER OR BATHE

Standard Precautions ☐ Handwashing ☐ Gloving ☐ Gowning ☐ Masking

Introductory Tasks ☐ Gather Equipment ☐ Identify/Introduce/Explain ☐ Provide Privacy

	Yes	No
8. Assist the resident out of bed and to the bathing area. Use a shower chair, if necessary.	___	___
9. Have the resident sit on a chair while you prepare the water.	___	___
10. For a bath, fill the tub halfway with water. The water temperature should be between 105° F and 110° F. For a shower, turn on the water and adjust the temperature until the water is comfortable. Test the water temperature with your elbow or the inner part of your wrist.	___	___
11. Help the resident remove the bathrobe and slippers. Assist the resident into the tub or shower. The shower chair can be wheeled right into the shower if the resident needs to sit down, but prefers a shower over a tub bath.	___	___
12. Explain how to use the signal cord. Ask the resident to signal when bathing is complete. Place the bathing supplies within reach.	___	___
13. Place a bath towel on the chair. Leave the room if the resident is strong enough to be left alone, but stay nearby. Follow the rules for your facility. Many facilities require a nursing assistant to remain in the room while residents bathe or shower.	___	___
14. Wash your hands.	___	___
15. Check the resident every five minutes. A resident should not remain in the tub or shower for more than 20 minutes.	___	___
16. Return when the resident signals. Knock before entering.	___	___
17. Help the resident out of the tub or shower and onto the chair.	___	___
18. Wrap the bath towels around the resident. Help the resident dry off.	___	___
19. Help the resident apply deodorant or antiperspirant and any other personal care products requested.	___	___
20. Provide a back massage.	___	___
21. Help the resident into clean clothes.	___	___
22. Help the resident return to his or her room.	___	___
23. Make the resident comfortable and provide for safety.	___	___
24. Gather all soiled linen and place it in the dirty laundry hamper.	___	___
25. Clean, replace, and store equipment for the next use. Discard disposable items.	___	___
26. Unscreen the resident.	___	___

	Yes	No
27. Clean the bathing area. Wash your hands.	___	___
28. Report any unusual observations to the supervisor.	___	___

Procedure Completed ______________________ **Date** ______________

Notes ____

____

____

PROCEDURE

OBRA SP

GIVING A FULL BED BATH

Standard Precautions ☐ Handwashing ☐ Gloving ☐ Gowning ☐ Masking

Introductory Tasks ☐ Gather Equipment ☐ Identify/Introduce/Explain ☐ Provide Privacy

	Yes	No
5. Line the over-bed table with paper towels. Place the supplies on it. Adjust the table to a comfortable working height.	___	___
6. Offer the bedpan or urinal. (Always wear gloves when in contact with bodily fluids.)	___	___
7. Put on clean gloves if the resident has any open lesions or wounds. Always wear gloves when providing perineal care.	___	___
8. Assist the resident with oral hygiene.	___	___
9. Remove the top linens and cover the resident with a bath blanket. Protect the resident's privacy.	___	___
10. Lower the head of the bed so the resident is lying flat. Give the resident at least one pillow to raise the head slightly.	___	___
11. Slip the resident's gown or pajamas off underneath the blanket. Place the soiled clothing in a dirty linen hamper.	___	___
12. Fill the wash basin with warm water. Water should be between 110° F and 115° F. Place a basin on the over-bed table.	___	___
13. Lower the side rail on the side nearest you.	___	___
14. Place a face towel over the resident's chest to keep the bath blanket dry.	___	___
15. Form a mitt around your hand with one of the wash cloths.	___	___
16. Wet the mitt. Wash the resident's eyes with water only. Wipe eyes from the inside corner toward the outside corner.	___	___

	Yes	No
17. Ask the resident if you should use soap on the face.	___	___
18. Rinse the washcloth and apply soap, if requested. Wash the face, ears, and neck.	___	___
19. Pat dry the skin using the towel on the resident's chest.	___	___
20. Place a bath towel under the resident's far arm. Wash, rinse, and pat dry the arm, shoulder, axilla, and hand.	___	___
21. Repeat for the other arm.	___	___
22. Apply deodorant or antiperspirant if requested.	___	___
23. Apply body lotion and powder as needed or requested.	___	___
24. Care for the hands and nails, if necessary. Place the hands in a wash basin to soak.	___	___
25. Place a bath towel over the resident's chest. Fold the bath blanket underneath down to the resident's waist.	___	___
26. Reach under the bath towel to wash, rinse, and pat dry the chest area.	___	___
27. Pull the bath blanket down to the pubic area. Wash, rinse, and pat dry the abdomen.	___	___
28. Pull the bath blanket over the resident's body. Slide the towel out from under the blanket.	___	___
29. Change the water if it is cool or soapy. *Raise the side rail before you leave the resident to change the water.*	___	___
30. Fold the bath blanket up to expose one entire leg. Place a bath towel under the leg.	___	___
31. Flex the knee. Wash the leg with long strokes. Put the bath basin on the towel and place the resident's foot in the basin. Use the orange stick to clean under the toenails.	___	___
32. Remove the basin and pat dry the leg, foot, and toes. Dry between the toes. Cover the leg.	___	___
33. Repeat for the other leg.	___	___
34. Change the bath water. *Raise the side rail before you leave the resident to change the water.*	___	___
35. Turn the resident onto the side away from you. Help the resident move his or her back close to you. Place a bath towel on the bed along the resident's back.	___	___
36. Wash the resident's back and buttocks with long, firm strokes. Rinse and pat dry.	___	___
37. Allow the resident to wash the perineal area. Adjust the over-bed table so the resident can comfortably reach the supplies. Place the signal cord in the resident's reach. Tell the resident to call when he or she is finished. Answer the call promptly.	___	___
38. If the resident is unable to clean the perineal area, you will assist or do so.	___	___
39. Give the resident a back rub. Perform range-of-motion exercises as ordered.	___	___
40. Put a clean gown, pajamas, or street clothes on the resident.	___	___
41. Place a towel over the resident's pillow. Comb or brush the hair.	___	___

	Yes	No
42. Make the bed and change the linens if the bedding is wet.	___	___
43. Lower the resident's bed. Raise the side rails.	___	___
44. Make the resident comfortable and provide for safety.	___	___
45. Gather all soiled linen and place it in the dirty laundry hamper.	___	___
46. Clean, replace, and store equipment for the next use. Discard disposable items.	___	___
47. Wipe off the over-bed table with the paper towels. Discard them.	___	___
48. Remove your gloves.	___	___
49. Unscreen the resident.	___	___
50. Wash your hands.	___	___
51. Report any unusual observations to the supervisor.	___	___

Procedure Completed ______________________________ **Date** ____________________

Notes ____

____

____

PROCEDURE

OBRA SP

GIVING A PARTIAL BED BATH

Standard Precautions ☐ Handwashing ☐ Gloving ☐ Gowning ☐ Masking

Introductory Tasks ☐ Gather Equipment ☐ Identify/Introduce/Explain ☐ Provide Privacy

	Yes	No
5. Line the over-bed table with paper towels. Place the supplies on it. Adjust the table to a comfortable working height.	___	___
6. Offer the bedpan or urinal. (Always wear gloves when in contact with bodily fluids.)	___	___
7. Put on gloves if the resident has any open lesions or wounds. Always wear gloves when providing perineal care.	___	___
8. Assist the resident with oral hygiene.	___	___
9. Remove the top linens and cover the resident with a bath blanket. Help the resident remove the hospital gown.	___	___
10. Raise the head of the bed so the resident can bathe comfortably. If he or she is able, help the resident sit on the side of the bed.	___	___

	Yes	No
11. Fill the wash basin with warm water. The water should be between 110° F and 115° F. Place the basin on the over-bed table.	___	___
12. Position the table so it is within easy reach of the resident.	___	___
13. Place the towels, soap, water, and washcloth within easy reach.	___	___
14. Tell the resident to wash as much as he or she is able. You will return to help with the rest.	___	___
15. Many facilities require the nursing assistant to stay during the bath. If not, place the signal cord in reach. Instruct the resident to call you when bathing is complete or if help is needed.	___	___
16. Wash your hands and leave the room, if appropriate.	___	___
17. Answer the call bell promptly. Ask what areas were not washed. Wash the areas the resident was unable to reach. Make sure the hands, face, axillae, buttocks, and perineum are clean and dry.	___	___
18. Give a back rub.	___	___
19. Help the resident apply deodorant or antiperspirant and put on a clean gown.	___	___
20. Apply body lotion or powder as needed or requested.	___	___
21. Place a towel over the resident's pillow. Comb or brush the hair.	___	___
22. Make the bed and change the linens if necessary.	___	___
23. Lower the bed. Raise the side rails.	___	___
24. Make the resident comfortable and provide for safety.	___	___
25. Gather all soiled linen and place it in the dirty linen hamper.	___	___
26. Clean, replace, and store equipment for the next use. Discard disposable items.	___	___
27. Wipe off the over-bed table with the paper towels. Discard them.	___	___
28. Unscreen the resident.	___	___
29. Wash your hands.	___	___
30. Report any unusual observations to the supervisor.	___	___

Procedure Completed ________________________ **Date** ____________________

Notes ____

____

____

PROCEDURE

OBRA

GIVING A WHIRLPOOL BATH

Standard Precautions	☐ Handwashing	☐ Gloving	☐ Gowning	☐ Masking
Introductory Tasks	☐ Gather Equipment	☐ Identify/Introduce/Explain	☐ Provide Privacy	

Step	Yes	No
11. Help the resident undress. Cover him or her with a bath blanket.	___	___
12. Position the resident in a whirlpool chair. Secure the straps. Take the resident to the tub.	___	___
13. Place the bath towels over the resident. Remove and fold the bath blanket.	___	___
14. Some whirlpool baths open on the side so the resident sits as if in a chair. Others have lifts with slings. Step on the "up" pedal to engage the chair. Make sure that both pins are locked into the arm slots. Secure the safety latches.	___	___
15. Raise the seat to its maximum height. Rotate the seat 90 degrees so the resident is facing you. Guide the chair to the tub edge so the resident is over the tub edge and parallel to the tub.	___	___
16. Guide the resident's feet over the tub edge and toward the bottom of the tub.	___	___
17. Lower the resident into the tub by gently pressing down on the pedal or electronic control. The water should reach the resident's chest.	___	___
18. Press the turbine button to turn on the whirlpool. The whirlpool should run for five minutes.	___	___
19. After the whirlpool stops, put on your gloves. Wash the resident's face and upper body.	___	___
20. Step on the "up" pedal until the resident's feet are level with the whirlpool. Dry the upper body.	___	___
21. Raise the seat to the maximum height. Pull the chair and the resident toward you, as you lift the resident's feet out of the tub.	___	___
22. Dry the legs and feet.	___	___
23. Cover the resident with a bath blanket.	___	___
24. Lift the safety latch on the whirlpool chair.	___	___
25. Slowly lower the lift until the whirlpool chair is flat on the floor.	___	___
26. Remove your gloves. Help the resident dress. Gather all the soiled linen and place it in the dirty linen hamper.	___	___
27. Return the resident to the room. Help with grooming.	___	___
28. Make the bed and change linens, if necessary.	___	___
29. Make the resident comfortable and provide for safety.	___	___
30. Unscreen the resident.	___	___

	Yes	No
31. Wash your hands.	___	___
32. Return to the tub room and clean the tub according to the manufacturer's directions.	___	___
33. Clean, replace, and store equipment for the next use. Discard disposable items.	___	___
34. Report any unusual observations to the supervisor.	___	___

Procedure Completed ______________________ **Date** ______________________

Notes ____

PROCEDURE

OBRA SP

HELPING NONAMBULATORY RESIDENTS SHAVE

Standard Precautions ☐ Handwashing ☐ Gloving ☐ Gowning ☐ Masking

Introductory Tasks ☐ Gather Equipment ☐ Identify/Introduce/Explain ☐ Provide Privacy

	Yes	No
5. Position the over-bed table so it is at a comfortable working height. Assemble the equipment so you or the resident can easily reach it.	___	___
6. Raise the head of the bed to the highest position. Make the resident comfortable.	___	___
7. Drape the resident's chest with a large towel.	___	___
8. Position the mirror so the resident can see his face.	___	___
9. If the resident uses an electric razor, make sure the razor is clean. Show the resident how to hold the razor and how to turn it on and off. Stay with the resident as he shaves. Make sure the resident does not miss any areas.	___	___
10. If a resident is using a disposable razor, fill the wash basin with warm water. Use a warm washcloth to dampen the face and soften the hair. Help the resident apply the shaving cream or gel.	___	___
11. Help the resident shave himself. Clean the razor in the wash basin whenever hair or shaving cream accumulates. Never leave a resident alone when he is shaving.	___	___
12. When the resident is done shaving, provide a clean, warm washcloth so he can wipe his face. Dry his face thoroughly.	___	___

	Yes	No
13. If the skin gets nicked, apply pressure directly over the spot with a gauze pad. Report the incident to the supervisor.	___	___
14. Help the resident apply after-shave lotion if he wishes.	___	___
15. Dispose of the razor in the sharps container.	___	___
16. Clean the supplies and store them for the next use.	___	___
17. Place dirty linens in a dirty linen hamper.	___	___
18. Remove your gloves.	___	___
19. Make the resident comfortable and provide for safety.	___	___
20. Unscreen the resident.	___	___
21. Wash your hands.	___	___
22. Report any unusual observations to the supervisor.	___	___

Procedure Completed ______________________ **Date** ______________

Notes ____

____

____

PROCEDURE

OBRA SP

SHAVING A DEPENDENT RESIDENT

Standard Precautions ☐ Handwashing ☐ Gloving ☐ Gowning ☐ Masking

Introductory Tasks ☐ Gather Equipment ☐ Identify/Introduce/Explain ☐ Provide Privacy

	Yes	No
5. Position the over-bed tray so it is at a comfortable working height. Assemble the equipment so you or the resident can easily reach it.	___	___
6. Raise the head of the bed to the highest position. Make the resident comfortable.	___	___
7. Drape the resident's chest with a large towel.	___	___
8. Position the mirror so the resident can see his face.	___	___
9. If the resident uses an electric razor, make sure the razor is clean. Shave the face, including the chin and neck area.	___	___
10. If the resident uses a disposable razor, fill the wash basin with warm water. Use a washcloth to dampen the face.	___	___

	Yes	No
11. Apply the shaving cream or gel on the face, including the neck area.	___	___
12. Start in front of one ear. Hold the skin tight. Bring the razor down the cheek toward the chin. Repeat until the shaving cream lather is gone.	___	___
13. Shave the area between the nose and the upper lip by moving the razor in short, downward strokes. Clean the razor in the wash basin whenever hair or shaving cream accumulates.	___	___
14. Ask the resident to raise his chin. Shave the neck area by bringing the razor up toward the chin.	___	___
15. Use a clean, warm washcloth to wash the face and neck. Dry thoroughly.	___	___
16. Apply after-shave lotion, if he wishes.	___	___
17. If the skin has been nicked, apply pressure directly over the spot with a gauze pad. Report the incident to the charge nurse.	___	___
18. Dispose of the razor in the sharps container.	___	___
19. Clean the supplies and store them for the next use.	___	___
20. Place dirty linens in a dirty linen hamper.	___	___
21. Remove your gloves.	___	___
22. Make the resident comfortable and provide for safety.	___	___
23. Unscreen the resident.	___	___
24. Wash your hands.	___	___
25. Report any unusual observations to the supervisor and, to protect yourself, document the report on the back of the ADL flow sheet. Have the supervisor or charge nurse initial your report.	___	___

Procedure Completed ______________________ **Date** ______________________

Notes ____

____

____

PROCEDURE

OBRA SP

CHANGING A HOSPITAL GOWN

Standard Precautions ☐ Handwashing ☐ Gloving ☐ Gowning ☐ Masking

Introductory Tasks ☐ Gather Equipment ☐ Identify/Introduce/Explain ☐ Provide Privacy

	Yes	No
5. Ask the resident to turn to the side so you can untie the gown. If the resident cannot turn, reach under the neck to untie the gown. If the resident has weakness on one side, remove the gown from the stronger side first.	___	___
6. Loosen the soiled gown around the body.	___	___
7. Unfold the clean gown and lay it over the resident's chest.	___	___
8. Remove one sleeve at a time, leaving the old gown draped over the resident's body.	___	___
9. Slide each arm through a sleeve of the clean gown. If the resident cannot move an arm, take that hand in your hand and slide it through the sleeve. Always place the weaker arm in a sleeve first, then place the stronger arm in the other sleeve.	___	___
10. Remove the soiled gown from under the clean gown.	___	___
11. Correctly position the clean gown and fasten the ties.	___	___
12. Place the soiled gown in the dirty linen hamper.	___	___
13. Make the resident comfortable and provide for safety.	___	___
14. Unscreen the resident.	___	___
15. Wash your hands.	___	___
16. Report any unusual observations to the supervisor.	___	___

Procedure Completed ______________________________ **Date** ______________________

Notes ____

____

____

PROCEDURE

OBRA SP

HELPING A NONAMBULATORY RESIDENT DRESS

Standard Precautions	☐ Handwashing	☐ Gloving	☐ Gowning	☐ Masking
Introductory Tasks	☐ Gather Equipment	☐ Identify/Introduce/Explain	☐ Provide Privacy	

Step	Yes	No
4. Check the resident's clothing to make sure it is clean and in good repair.	___	___
5. Remove the clothing the resident is wearing.	___	___
6. First put on the resident's underwear. To put on underpants, position the resident on his or her back. Guide the feet through the leg openings. Pull the underpants up the legs and position the elastic at waist level.	___	___
7. Use the same technique to dress a resident in slacks or panty hose.	___	___
8. Put on each sock. Make sure the toes are correctly aligned and the heel of the sock is positioned correctly on the foot.	___	___
9. Put on the resident's shoes or slippers, as the resident requests.	___	___
10. Put a brassiere on female residents. Slide her arms through the bra straps. Adjust the cups to fit over the breasts and adjust the shoulder straps.	___	___
11. Close the hooks in back or in front as required. You can put the bra on backwards by closing the hooks in front and rotating the bra around the body if you find it easier. Then guide the resident's arms through the straps.	___	___
12. Put on the resident's shirt and/or undershirt. If residents can dress themselves, they should put their arms through the sleeves of the garment. You can then help pull the garment over their head. If the resident cannot dress himself or herself, pull the garment over his or her head. Place one arm at a time through each sleeve. Place the weak arm through first, then the stronger arm. Adjust the garment to fit the body. Button, zip, or snap the shirt as needed.	___	___
13. If a female resident chooses to wear a dress, place the dress over her head. Place the resident's arms through each sleeve. Adjust the dress over the resident's body and button or zip the dress.	___	___
14. Make the resident comfortable and provide for safety.	___	___
15. Place the dirty clothes in a dirty linen hamper.	___	___
16. Wash your hands.	___	___
17. Report any unusual observations to the supervisor.	___	___

Procedure Completed ______________________ Date ______________

Notes ____

____

____

PROCEDURE

OBRA

HELPING A RESIDENT UNDRESS

	Yes	No
1. Assist the resident to a comfortable position. Open all the clothing. For example, unzip a dress, unbutton the shirt, or unzip the trousers.	___	___
2. Remove a dress or shirt by gently moving the garment up the body. Guide each arm out of the garment. Pull the garment over the head. If requested, remove a female resident's bra. Open the hooks and slip off the bra.	___	___
3. If you are dressing the resident in pajamas or a hospital gown, put the garments on now. You do not want to leave the resident uncovered.	___	___
4. Help the resident lie down and remove shoes and socks.	___	___
5. Pull slacks or panty hose gently down the legs from the waist.	___	___
6. Remove underpants. Replace with clean underpants if the resident requests them.	___	___
7. Make the resident comfortable and provide for safety.	___	___
8. Place the dirty clothes in the dirty linen hamper. Fold or hang clean garments in the closet.	___	___
9. Wash your hands.	___	___

Procedure Completed ______________________ Date ______________

Notes ____

____

____

PROCEDURE

OBRA SP

CLEANING THE FEMALE PERINEAL AREA

Standard Precautions ☐ Handwashing ☐ Gloving ☐ Gowning ☐ Masking

Introductory Tasks ☐ Gather Equipment ☐ Identify/Introduce/Explain ☐ Provide Privacy

	Yes	No
5. Cover the resident with the bath blanket. Move the top linens to the bottom of the bed.	___	___
6. Position the resident on her back. Place the bed protector under her hips.	___	___
7. Ask the resident whether she is able to clean her perineal area.	___	___
8. Fill the basin with warm water. Place the basin on the over-bed table, along with the soap or perineal wash, washcloth or disposable wipes, and the towel.	___	___
9. Undrape only the area between the resident's legs.	___	___
10. Put on gloves. If the resident is able to clean herself, give her privacy. Place the signal cord in her reach and leave the room. Return in a couple of minutes.	___	___
11. If the resident is unable to clean herself, raise the bed to a comfortable position for you to work. Help the resident flex her knees and spread her legs.	___	___
12. Wet the washcloth and make a mitt around your hand. (Some facilities use a perineal wash solution instead of soap.) Use one gloved hand to separate the vulva. With the other gloved hand, wipe the pubic area from the front to the back using single strokes. Wipe down the center first, then wipe each side. Rinse the washcloth often. Wipe the inner labia. Rinse the washcloth. Clean and rinse the inner part of the vulva.	___	___
13. Rinse and dry the area thoroughly.	___	___
14. Turn the resident away from you. Expose and cleanse the anal area. Rinse the washcloth often. Continue wiping until the area is clean. *Always wipe from front to back.*	___	___
15. Dry the anal area.	___	___
16. Return the resident to her back.	___	___
17. Remove and dispose of the bed protector.	___	___
18. Cover the resident with the bed sheet.	___	___
19. Make the resident comfortable and provide for safety.	___	___
20. Empty the dirty water into the toilet. Place the dirty linens in the dirty linen hamper. Clean and store equipment for the next use.	___	___
21. Remove your gloves. Wash your hands.	___	___
22. Unscreen the resident.	___	___
23. Report any unusual observations to the supervisor.	___	___

Procedure Completed ______________________ **Date** ______________

Notes ____

____

____

PROCEDURE

GIVING A VAGINAL DOUCHE

Standard Precautions ☐ Handwashing ☐ Gloving ☐ Gowning ☐ Masking

Introductory Tasks ☐ Gather Equipment ☐ Identify/Introduce/Explain ☐ Provide Privacy

	Yes	**No**
5. Offer the bedpan to the resident and encourage her to urinate. Her bladder should be empty.	___	___
6. Put on your gloves. Empty the bedpan. Clean and store it.	___	___
7. Remove gloves and wash your hands.	___	___
8. Warm the irrigation solution to 105° F. If the solution is prepackaged, place the package in a basin of warm water to warm it.	___	___
9. Position the resident on her back. Place the waterproof bed protector under her hips. Drape the resident with the bath blanket so only the area between her legs is exposed.	___	___
10. Put on clean gloves. Perform perineal care.	___	___
11. Position the resident on the bedpan. Hang the irrigation solution on the IV pole. Remove the cover from the douche container. Release the clamp to start the flow of the irrigation solution. Let some solution run over the perineal area.	___	___
12. Tell the resident that you are going to insert the douche tip.	___	___
13. Insert the tip 3 to 4 inches into the vagina. Release the clamp to start the flow. Hold the douche bag 12 inches above the vagina for proper flow.	___	___
14. Rotate the tip often. Use all the solution.	___	___
15. Remove the douche tip from the vagina. The remaining solution will drain from the vagina into the bedpan.	___	___
16. Place the tubing in the irrigation container. Remove the douching equipment.	___	___
17. Remove the bedpan. Thoroughly dry the perineal area. Dispose of the waterproof bed protector.	___	___
18. Cover the resident with the top covers and make her comfortable. Provide for safety.	___	___

	Yes	No
19. Empty the contents of the bedpan in the toilet. Place the dirty linens in the dirty linen hamper. Clean and store equipment for the next use.	___	___
20. Remove your gloves. Wash your hands.	___	___
21. Unscreen the resident.	___	___
22. Report any unusual observations to the supervisor.	___	___

Procedure Completed ______________________ **Date** ______________________

Notes ____

____

____

PROCEDURE

OBRA SP

CLEANING THE MALE PERINEAL AREA

Standard Precautions ☐ Handwashing ☐ Gloving ☐ Gowning ☐ Masking

Introductory Tasks ☐ Gather Equipment ☐ Identify/Introduce/Explain ☐ Provide Privacy

	Yes	No
5. Cover the resident with the bath blanket. Move the top linens to the bottom of the bed.	___	___
6. Position the resident on his back. Place the bed protector under his hips.	___	___
7. Ask the resident whether he is able to clean his perineal area.	___	___
8. Fill the basin with warm water (105° F). Place the basin on the over-bed table, along with the soap, washcloth or disposable wipes, and the towel.	___	___
9. Undrape only the area between the resident's legs.	___	___
10. Put on gloves. If the resident is able to clean himself, give him privacy. Place the signal cord within his reach and leave the room. Return in a couple of minutes.	___	___
11. If the resident is unable to clean himself, raise the bed to a comfortable position for you to work. Help the resident flex his knees and spread his legs.	___	___
12. Wet the washcloth and make a mitt around your hand. Use one gloved hand to retract the foreskin if the resident is uncircumcised. Grasp the penis.	___	___
13. Wash the penis using a circular motion from the bottom of the shaft towards the top (urethra opening). Rinse the washcloth often. Rinse the area. Return the foreskin to its natural position. Rinse the area.	___	___
14. Cleanse the scrotum.	___	___

	Yes	No
15. Rinse and dry the area thoroughly.	___	___
16. Turn the resident away from you. Expose and cleanse the anal area. Rinse the washcloth often. Continue wiping until the area is clean. *Always wipe from front to back.*	___	___
17. Dry the anal area.	___	___
18. Return the resident to his back.	___	___
19. Remove and dispose of the bed protector.	___	___
20. Cover the resident with the top covers.	___	___
21. Make the resident comfortable and provide for safety.	___	___
22. Empty the dirty water into the toilet. Place the dirty linens in the dirty linen hamper. Clean and store equipment for the next use.	___	___
23. Remove your gloves. Wash your hands.	___	___
24. Unscreen the resident.	___	___
25. Report any unusual observations to the supervisor.	___	___

Procedure Completed ______________________________ **Date** ____________________

Notes ____

____

____

PROCEDURE

APPLYING LOTION TO PREVENT PRESSURE SORES

Standard Precautions ☐ Handwashing ☐ Gloving ☐ Gowning ☐ Masking

Introductory Tasks ☐ Gather Equipment ☐ Identify/Introduce/Explain ☐ Provide Privacy

	Yes	No
5. Position the over-bed tray so it is at a comfortable working height. Assemble the equipment.	___	___
6. If the resident already has pressure sores, put on gloves.	___	___
7. Expose the area that you will work with first. Drape the rest of the body with the bath blanket.	___	___
8. Put some lotion in your hands and rub your hands together to warm the lotion.	___	___
9. Massage the lotion into the skin in a circular motion. Work around an infected area, not directly on it. Massage all the dry skin in the area.	___	___

	Yes	No
10. Gently pat dry excess lotion with a bath towel.	___	___
11. Repeat Steps 7 through 10 on each area that shows signs of developing a pressure sore, as well as on all bony areas of the skin. Move the draping around the resident so only the area you are working on is exposed.	___	___
12. Redress the resident. Reposition the resident. Cushion areas that are at risk for pressure sores.	___	___
13. Make the resident comfortable and provide for safety.	___	___
14. Place the dirty linens in the dirty linen hamper. Clean and store the lotion container for the next use.	___	___
15. Remove your gloves. Wash your hands.	___	___
16. Unscreen the resident.	___	___
17. Report any unusual observations to the supervisor.	___	___

Procedure Completed ______________________ **Date** ______________________

Notes ____

____

____

PROCEDURE

OBRA SP

CLEANING AND TRIMMING FINGERNAILS

Standard Precautions ☐ Handwashing ☐ Gloving ☐ Gowning ☐ Masking

Introductory Tasks ☐ Gather Equipment ☐ Identify/Introduce/Explain ☐ Provide Privacy

	Yes	No
5. Position the over-bed table so it is at a comfortable working height. Assemble your equipment.	___	___
6. Help the resident to a bedside chair. Place the signal cord within reach.	___	___
7. If a resident is wearing nail polish and wants it changed, remove the nail polish. Put a small amount of nail polish remover on a cotton ball and gently rub each nail.	___	___
8. Place a towel or bathmat on the floor under the resident's feet. Adjust the over-bed table so it is at a comfortable height in front of the resident.	___	___
9. Line the over-bed table with paper towels. Place the emesis basin on the table. Fill the basin with warm water. Place the resident's ten fingers in the basin.	___	___

	Yes	No
10. Let the hands soak for at least five minutes. Rewarm the water if necessary.	___	___
11. Remove the resident's hands from the basin. Dry the hands thoroughly with the towel.	___	___
12. Use the orange stick or a towel to push back the cuticles, if this is facility policy. (Pushing the cuticles back is now avoided in many places.) Clean under each nail.	___	___
13. Clip fingernails straight across. Do not cut too close to the skin.	___	___
14. Shape nails with the emery board. Wash the resident's hands to remove any debris.	___	___
15. Massage the resident's hands with lotion. Apply nail polish if the resident requests it.	___	___
16. Help the resident return to bed.	___	___
17. Make the resident comfortable and provide for safety.	___	___
18. Clean and store the equipment for the next use. Discard disposable equipment. Remove soiled linens.	___	___
19. Unscreen the resident.	___	___
20. Wash your hands.	___	___
21. Report any unusual observations to the supervisor.	___	___

Procedure Completed ______________________ **Date** ______________________

Notes ____

____

____

PROCEDURE

OBRA SP

GIVING A BACK RUB

Standard Precautions ☐ Handwashing ☐ Gloving ☐ Gowning ☐ Masking

Introductory Tasks ☐ Gather Equipment ☐ Identify/Introduce/Explain ☐ Provide Privacy

	Yes	No
5. Raise the bed to a comfortable working height. Lower the side rail on your side.	___	___
6. Position the resident flat on the bed in a prone position, or in a side-lying position with the back toward you.	___	___

	Yes	No
7. Expose the back, shoulders, and the top of the buttocks. Cover the rest of the body with the bath blanket.	___	___
8. Warm the lotion under warm running water or rub some lotion between your hands.	___	___
9. Explain to the resident that the lotion may feel wet and cool.	___	___
10. Make long, firm strokes with both hands. Always keep at least one hand on the resident's back during the back rub. Apply more lotion as needed.	___	___
11. Begin at the buttocks. Stroke in an upward motion toward the shoulders. Complete a circle at the shoulders and massage the upper arms. Bring your hands back down the back, one hand on each side, in a circular motion. Complete a circle at the buttocks and repeat the cycle for 3 to 5 minutes.	___	___
12. Massage bony areas and pressure spots using a circular motion with the fingers.	___	___
13. Make long, firm stokes to end the back rub. Tell the resident you are finishing.	___	___
14. Gently pat dry any excess lotion with the bath towel.	___	___
15. Refasten the resident's gown. Remove the bath blanket and cover the resident.	___	___
16. Raise the side rail and make the resident comfortable. Provide for safety.	___	___
17. Clean and store lotion for the next use. Remove soiled linens.	___	___
18. Unscreen the resident.	___	___
19. Wash your hands.	___	___
20. Report any unusual observations to the supervisor.	___	___

Procedure Completed ______________________________ **Date** ______________________

Notes ____

____

____

PROCEDURE

OBRA SP

CARING FOR THE RESIDENT'S EYEGLASSES

Standard Precautions ☐ Handwashing ☐ Gloving ☐ Gowning ☐ Masking

Introductory Tasks ☐ Gather Equipment ☐ Identify/Introduce/Explain ☐ Provide Privacy

	Yes	No
5. Remove the glasses from the resident, touching only the frames.	___	___
6. Clean the glasses with cool running water and rinse with a cleaning solution.	___	___
7. Dry them with a cloth (lint-free, if available). Paper products can scratch plastic lenses.	___	___
8. Place the eyeglasses in an eyeglass case or return them to the resident.	___	___
9. Make the resident comfortable and provide for safety.	___	___
10. Unscreen the resident.	___	___
11. Wash your hands.	___	___

Procedure Completed ______________________ **Date** ______________

Notes ____

____

____

PROCEDURE

SP

CARING FOR AN ARTIFICIAL EYE

Standard Precautions ☐ Handwashing ☐ Gloving ☐ Gowning ☐ Masking

Introductory Tasks ☐ Gather Equipment ☐ Identify/Introduce/Explain ☐ Provide Privacy

	Yes	No
5. Assist the resident into bed. Performing this procedure with the resident in bed helps prevent damage to the artificial eye if it accidentally falls.	___	___
6. Clean the outside of the eye. Use a cotton ball to wipe from the inner corner to the outer corner. Use each cotton ball for one wipe on one eye.	___	___

	Yes	No
7. Ask the resident to remove the artificial eye. If you have to remove it, carefully depress the lower eyelid with your thumb. Lift the upper eyelid with your forefinger. The eye should slide out into your hand.	___	___
8. Place the eye in the eyecup on top of a piece of gauze. Let it soak in water.	___	___
9. Clean the eye socket using a normal saline solution or warm water and cotton balls. Remove any debris and encrustation. Gently dry the area around the eye.	___	___
10. Carry the eyecup to the sink. Rinse out the sink. Fill the sink halfway with warm water, in case you accidentally drop the eye. Place a washcloth on the bottom of the sink as an added precaution.	___	___
11. Rinse the eye under lukewarm running water. Discard the water and gauze from the eyecup. Place the slightly moist eye on a new piece of gauze in the eyecup.	___	___
12. If the resident is not going to wear the eye, put some water in the eyecup to store it.	___	___
13. Wash your hands. Return to the resident to insert the eye. If the resident is able to insert the eye, have the resident wash his or her hands.	___	___
14. To insert the eye, depress the lower eyelid. Raise the upper lid with your forefinger. With your other hand, insert the eye. The eye should settle in place.	___	___
15. Make the resident comfortable and provide for safety.	___	___
16. Clean and store equipment for the next use.	___	___
17. Unscreen the resident.	___	___
18. Wash your hands.	___	___
19. Report any unusual observations to the supervisor.	___	___

Procedure Completed ______________________ **Date** ______________________

Notes ____

____

____

PROCEDURE

OBRA SP

REMOVING AND INSERTING A HEARING AID

Standard Precautions ☐ Handwashing ☐ Gloving ☐ Gowning ☐ Masking

Introductory Tasks ☐ Gather Equipment ☐ Identify/Introduce/Explain ☐ Provide Privacy

	Yes	**No**
Inserting the Hearing Aid:		
5. Check the resident's ear for wax buildup or anything unusual. Turn the hearing aid off.	___	___
6. If the resident is able, allow him or her to insert the hearing aid.	___	___
7. If you are inserting the hearing aid, place the hearing aid over the resident's ear, if appropriate, with the ear mold piece hanging free.	___	___
8. Adjust the hearing aid behind the ear.	___	___
9. Gently insert the ear mold into the ear canal. Gently twist the ear mold into the curve of the ear. Push up and in with one hand. Use your other hand to pull gently on the earlobe.	___	___
10. Turn the hearing aid on and adjust the volume to a comfortable level.	___	___
11. If the resident complains that the hearing aid is uncomfortable, it may need to be refitted. Report this to the supervisor.	___	___
Removing the Hearing Aid:		
12. Turn off the hearing aid.	___	___
13. Gently pull on the upper ear to loosen the outer portion of the hearing aid.	___	___
14. Lift the ear mold up and out.	___	___
15. Remove the batteries before storing the hearing aid in its case in a safe place. Make sure the case is labeled with the resident's name.	___	___
16. Make the resident comfortable and provide for safety.	___	___
17. Unscreen the resident.	___	___
18. Wash your hands.	___	___
19. Report any unusual observations to the supervisor.	___	___

Procedure Completed ______________________ **Date** ______________

Notes ____

____

____

CHAPTER 19

ASSISTING THE ELDERLY IN LONG-TERM CARE

STUDY OBJECTIVES

Some elderly are able to maintain active lives. Others may live in facilities that provide long-term care. Residents should be encouraged to remain as active as possible, both physically and mentally. Aging lessens the intensity of the senses. It also lessens the ability of organs to function. Psychologically and socially, aging brings the changes that go along with the loss of friends and family, sometimes resulting in depression. OBRA requires long-term care facilities to care for residents in a way that promotes dignity, self-esteem, and physical, psychological, spiritual, and emotional well-being.

- Helping ambulatory residents exercise usually includes encouraging daily walks and participation in group exercise. Residents on bed rest can exercise their arms and legs if the doctor approves such a regimen. Residents can exercise in wheelchairs by moving their arms and legs.
- The physical changes of aging usually include slowing down of organ function and lessening of the intensity of the senses. Skin is drier.
- The psychological and social changes of aging usually include loss of family and friends, ending of career, loss of independence, change in personal relationships, and adjustment to a new family role and environment.
- OBRA regulations require facilities to maintain certain standards and to promote the dignity and self-esteem of residents.
- Nursing assistants provide whatever personal care residents with mental illness require. They also help such residents maintain a reality orientation.

KNOW YOUR TERMS

In the space provided, write the letter of the definition that best fits the numbered term.

__ 1. atrophy	a. An order to have a patient stay in bed without getting up at all for a period of time.
__ 2. contracture	b. A wasting away of (said of tissues, a body part, or a whole body).
__ 3. strict bed rest	c. A muscle shortening due to spasm or loss of muscular control.

TEST YOUR KNOWLEDGE

Write the word(s) that best completes the statement.

1. Muscle _____________ occurs when muscles decrease in size and waste away.
2. _____________ and _____________ are terms referring to people in the later years of their lives.
3. Arteries and veins narrow as the body ages, thereby _____________ blood flow.
4. In the aging process, the skin becomes _____________.
5. Hormones released by the endocrine system _____________ as one ages.
6. A _____________-_____________ diet encourages bowel regularity.
7. _____________ _____________ is a technique based on constant repetition of information to disoriented residents.
8. Never _____________ an agitated resident.
9. _____________ is the most common mental disorder in the elderly.
10. _____________ residents are suspicious and distrustful.

THINK ABOUT THE ISSUES

1. OBRA regulations protect the rights of the elderly in long-term care. Do you think such regulations are necessary? Why or why not?
2. List some ways nursing assistants can help care for patients with mental disorders.

CHAPTER 20

VITAL SIGNS AND MEASUREMENTS

STUDY OBJECTIVES

Vital signs (pulse, respiration, temperature, and blood pressure) are indicators of the statc of a person's health. Height and weight measure how well a person is maintaining bone structure and nutrition.

- Normal temperature ranges vary depending on the individual. Medication can affect a temperature reading.
- Temperature can be measured in several different ways with different thermometers.
- Pulse rates provide an overall indication of how well a patient's circulatory system is functioning. Pulses can be measured at a number of different points on the body.
- Respiration is observed for rate and sound. Abnormal respiration can indicate serious problems.
- Blood pressure is a measure of the force of the blood flow exerted against the walls of the artery. Blood pressure is measured with any of several instruments.
- Height and weight can be measured on an upright scale, an in-bed scale, or on a wheelchair scale.

KNOW YOUR TERMS

In the space provided, write the letter of the definition that best fits the numbered term.

__ 1. apical pulse	a. A condition with a heartbeat below 60 beats per minute.
__ 2. apnea	b. The part of the blood pressure that measures the rhythmic dilation of the heart cavities as they fill with blood.
__ 3. blood pressure	c. The rhythmic throbbing caused by the contractions of the heart muscle.
__ 4. body temperature	d. Shortness of breath.
__ 5. bradycardia	e. An instrument for measuring body temperature.
__ 6. diastolic pressure	f. The pulse measured 2 to 3 inches to the left of the sternum.
__ 7. dyspnea	g. Failure to breathe.
__ 8. hypotension	h. Rapid beating of the heart.
__ 9. pulse	i. Important indicators of how well the body systems are functioning, including pulse, temperature, respiration, and blood pressure.
__10. pulse deficit	j. An instrument for listening to body sounds.
__11. radial pulse	k. The degree of heat or cold of the body.
__12. sphygmomanometer	l. The pulse measured at the wrist.
__13. stethoscope	m. The measurement of the contractions of the heart.
__14. systolic pressure	n. A measure of the pressure of blood upon the walls of the arteries and veins.
__15. tachycardia	o. An instrument for measuring blood pressure using a cuff, bulb, and a gauge.
__16. thermometer	p. Low blood pressure.
__17. vital signs	q. The difference between an apical and radial pulse.

TEST YOUR KNOWLEDGE

Write the word(s) that best completes the statement.

1. An ______________ thermometer measures a person's temperature in the mouth or under the arm.
2. A ______________ thermometer measures a person's temperature in the ear.
3. The ______________ ______________ measures the pressure that can be felt in the artery every time the heart beats.
4. The normal pulse rate for a newborn is ______________ than the one for an adolescent.

5. A _____________ pulse is measured at the wrist.
6. A _____________ is a device for listening to sounds in the body.
7. The process of breathing in and out is called _____________.
8. A _____________ is a device for measuring blood pressure.
9. _____________ pressure measures the force the heart exerts when it pumps blood out.
10. _____________ pressure measures the amount of pressure in the arteries between heartbeats.

▲ THINK ABOUT THE ISSUES

1. Why do you think it is necessary to take patients' vital signs?
2. If a patient refuses to eat and is losing weight, do you think the doctor should force-feed the patient? Why or why not?

▲ CHECK YOUR SKILLS

In the following procedure checklists, check each task box that applies and answer yes or no to each step you have completed. If possible, have your instructor sign off when you have completed a procedure.

PROCEDURE

OBRA

READING A GLASS THERMOMETER

	Yes	No
1. Pick up the thermometer and hold it at the stem end, using only your thumb and the tips of your fingers.	___	___
2. Bring the thermometer to eye level.	___	___
3. Turn the thermometer until the side with the printed scale is facing you.	___	___
4. Slowly rotate the thermometer until you can see the mercury inside the tube.	___	___
5. Look at the scale and read the measurement. Whether you are using a Fahrenheit or Centigrade thermometer, your reading should be to the nearest two-tenths of a degree.	___	___
6. Write down the temperature in your notebook or on a form, according to the facility's policy.	___	___

Procedure Completed ______________________________ **Date** ______________________

Notes ____

____

____

PROCEDURE

OBRA SP

MEASURING ORAL TEMPERATURE WITH A GLASS THERMOMETER

Standard Precautions ☐ Handwashing ☐ Gloving ☐ Gowning ☐ Masking

Introductory Tasks ☐ Gather Equipment ☐ Identify/Introduce/Explain ☐ Provide Privacy

	Yes	No
6. Hold the thermometer at the stem end.	___	___
7. Run cold water over the thermometer if it has been soaking in a disinfectant.	___	___
8. Gently dry the thermometer with tissues, starting at the stem and working toward the bulb.	___	___
9. Check the thermometer for cracks or chips.	___	___
10. Shake down the thermometer to below 95° Fahrenheit by holding it firmly and then snapping your wrist downward.	___	___
11. Slide a plastic sleeve over the thermometer.	___	___
12. Insert the bulb end of the thermometer under the patient's tongue.	___	___
13. Have the patient close the lips to help hold the thermometer in place.	___	___
14. Wait 3 to 5 minutes.	___	___
15. Gently grasp the end of the thermometer and remove it from the patient's mouth.	___	___
16. Remove the plastic sleeve. Be careful not to touch the bulb end.	___	___
17. Read the thermometer and record the reading according to facility policy.	___	___
18. Rinse under cool water, wash, and dry the thermometer.	___	___
19. Shake down the thermometer.	___	___
20. Soak the thermometer in the thermometer holder with disinfectant solution.	___	___
21. Check to make sure the patient is comfortable and place the signal light within reach.	___	___
22. Unscreen the patient.	___	___
23. Wash your hands.	___	___
24. Report abnormal temperature readings to the nurse.	___	___

Procedure Completed ______________________ **Date** ______________

Notes ____

____

____

PROCEDURE

OBRA SP

MEASURING TEMPERATURE WITH A RECTAL THERMOMETER

Standard Precautions ☐ Handwashing ☐ Gloving ☐ Gowning ☐ Masking

Introductory Tasks ☐ Gather Equipment ☐ Identify/Introduce/Explain ☐ Provide Privacy

	Yes	No
6. Hold the thermometer at the stem end.	___	___
7. Run cold water over the thermometer if it has been soaking in a disinfectant.	___	___
8. Gently dry the thermometer with tissues, starting at the stem and working toward the bulb.	___	___
9. Check the thermometer for cracks or chips.	___	___
10. Shake down the thermometer to below 95° Fahrenheit by holding it firmly and then snapping your wrist downward.	___	___
11. Cover the thermometer with a plastic sleeve.	___	___
12. Place a small amount of water-soluble lubricant on a piece of toilet tissue. Lubricate the bulb end of the thermometer to ease insertion.	___	___
13. Ask the patient to lie on his or her side. Help the patient turn, if necessary. (If the patient is apprehensive, suggest he or she take a deep breath and slowly exhale as the thermometer is being inserted.)	___	___
14. Fold back just enough of the linens to expose the patient's buttocks.	___	___
15. With one hand, raise the upper buttock to expose the anus.	___	___
16. Using the other hand, gently insert the thermometer 1 inch into the rectum.	___	___
17. Hold the thermometer in place for 3 minutes.	___	___
18. Remove the thermometer from the patient's rectum.	___	___
19. Wipe the patient's anal area to remove the lubricant. Re-cover the patient's buttocks with the bed linens.	___	___
20. Remove the plastic sleeve. Place the used toilet tissue on a paper towel and place the thermometer on a clean paper towel.	___	___
21. Read the thermometer and record the reading. Place an "R" next to the reading to indicate that it was a rectal reading. Discard soiled toilet tissue into the toilet.	___	___
22. Shake down the thermometer.	___	___
23. Rinse the thermometer with cool water, wash, and dry it. Remove your gloves and discard them.	___	___
24. Soak the thermometer in the thermometer holder with disinfectant solution.	___	___
25. Place the signal light within reach and check to make sure the patient is comfortable.	___	___

	Yes	No
26. Unscreen the patient.	___	___
27. Wash your hands.	___	___
28. Report abnormal temperature readings to the nurse.	___	___

Procedure Completed ______________________ **Date** ______________

Notes ____

____

____

PROCEDURE

OBRA SP

MEASURING TEMPERATURE WITH TYMPANIC THERMOMETER

Standard Precautions ☐ Handwashing ☐ Gloving ☐ Gowning ☐ Masking

Introductory Tasks ☐ Gather Equipment ☐ Identify/Introduce/Explain ☐ Provide Privacy

	Yes	No
6. Place the cone-shaped end of the thermometer into a probe cover.	___	___
7. Ask the patient to position his or her head so the ear is in front of you.	___	___
8. Gently grasp the outer portion of the patient's earlobe and pull it up and back to allow easier access to the ear canal.	___	___
9. Insert the covered probe into the patient's ear canal, pointing the probe down and toward the front of the canal.	___	___
10. Leave the probe in place until you hear or see a signal from the probe. Some models flash a light when the measurement is finished. Other models sound a tone.	___	___
11. Remove the probe from the ear canal.	___	___
12. Read the probe and record the reading. Place a "T" next to the reading to indicate that it was a tympanic reading.	___	___
13. Remove and discard the probe cover.	___	___
14. Place the thermometer back in its battery charger.	___	___
15. Place the signal light within reach and check to make sure the patient is comfortable.	___	___
16. Unscreen the patient.	___	___
17. Wash your hands.	___	___
18. Report abnormal temperature readings to the nurse.	___	___

Procedure Completed ______________________ **Date** ______________

Notes ____

PROCEDURE

OBRA SP

MEASURING AN AXILLARY TEMPERATURE

Standard Precautions ☐ Handwashing ☐ Gloving ☐ Gowning ☐ Masking

Introductory Tasks ☐ Gather Equipment ☐ Identify/Introduce/Explain ☐ Provide Privacy

	Yes	No
6. Hold the thermometer at the stem end.	___	___
7. Run cold water over the thermometer if it has been soaking in a disinfectant.	___	___
8. Gently dry the thermometer with tissues, starting at the stem and working toward the bulb.	___	___
9. Check the thermometer for cracks or chips.	___	___
10. Shake down the thermometer to below 95° Fahrenheit by holding it firmly and then snapping your wrist downward.	___	___
11. Slide a plastic sleeve over the thermometer.	___	___
12. Assist the patient in removing an arm from his or her shirt or gown.	___	___
13. Pat the axilla gently with a towel.	___	___
14. Position the bulb end of the thermometer in the center of the axilla.	___	___
15. Ask the patient to hold the arm close to the body or place the arm over the chest to hold the thermometer in place.	___	___
16. Wait 10 minutes and then remove the thermometer.	___	___
17. Remove the plastic sleeve. Be careful not to touch the bulb end.	___	___
18. Read the thermometer and record the reading. Place an "A" next to the reading to indicate that it was an axillary reading.	___	___
19. Rinse, wash, and dry the thermometer.	___	___
20. Shake down the thermometer.	___	___
21. Soak the thermometer in the thermometer holder with disinfectant solution.	___	___
22. Place the signal light within reach and check to make sure the patient is comfortable.	___	___
23. Unscreen the patient.	___	___
24. Wash your hands.	___	___
25. Report abnormal temperature readings to the nurse.	___	___

Procedure Completed ______________________ Date ______________________

Notes ____

____

____

PROCEDURE

CLEANING GLASS THERMOMETERS

Standard Precautions ☐ Handwashing ☐ Gloving ☐ Gowning ☐ Masking

Introductory Tasks ☐ Gather Equipment ☐ Identify/Introduce/Explain ☐ Provide Privacy

	Yes	No
2. Lay the towel out on the counter alongside the sink.	___	___
3. Wash and dry the container that will be used to store the clean thermometers. Lay it on the towel, with the open side facing up.	___	___
4. When the container is dry, put a piece of gauze in the bottom of it.	___	___
5. Clean the sink with cleanser.	___	___
6. Place a clean washcloth in the bottom of the sink. In case you drop a thermometer, the washcloth will help prevent breakage.	___	___
7. Fill the sink one-third full of cool water.	___	___
8. Put on disposable gloves.	___	___
9. Turn on the cold water. Water flow should not be too strong.	___	___
10. Moisten a cotton ball and apply soap.	___	___
11. Pick up the thermometer, holding it by the stem end.	___	___
12. Clean the thermometer with the cotton ball, moving from the stem end to the bulb end.	___	___
13. Discard the cotton ball.	___	___
14. Dry the thermometer using a new cotton ball.	___	___
15. Check the thermometer for chips and cracks.	___	___
16. Turn off the faucet.	___	___
17. Fill a clean container about half full with disinfectant.	___	___
18. Place the clean thermometer in the container with the disinfectant.	___	___
19. Cover the container and label it with your initials, and the date and time of the cleaning.	___	___
20. Empty the liquid from the container that housed the soiled thermometer.	___	___
21. Squeeze the excess water out of the washcloth and place it in the laundry.	___	___

	Yes	No
22. Fill the sink half full with hot water and soap. Wash, rinse, and dry the container that held the soiled thermometer.	___	___
23. Remove the disposable gloves and discard them.	___	___
24. Clean up your work area.	___	___
25. Place the towel in the laundry.	___	___
26. Place a clean, 4 x 4 folded sponge in the bottom of a clean container.	___	___
27. After the thermometer has soaked in the container long enough to disinfect according to facility policy, remove the thermometer from the disinfectant.	___	___
28. Place the disinfected thermometer on the sponge in the clean container and cover.	___	___
29. Clean the dirty container with disinfectant and dry.	___	___
30. Store the container with the clean thermometer and the empty container in the appropriate locations for your facility.	___	___
31. Wash your hands.	___	___

Procedure Completed______________________ **Date**______________________

Notes____

____

____

PROCEDURE

USING A DISPOSABLE THERMOMETER

Standard Precautions ☐ Handwashing ☐ Gloving ☐ Gowning ☐ Masking

Introductory Tasks ☐ Gather Equipment ☐ Identify/Introduce/Explain ☐ Provide Privacy

	Yes	No
6. Take the protective covering off the thermometer.	___	___
7. Ask the patient to wet his or her lips to ease insertion.	___	___
8. Insert the narrow end of the thermometer under the patient's tongue.	___	___
9. Have the patient close the lips. This helps hold the thermometer in place.	___	___
10. Wait 45 seconds.	___	___
11. Gently grasp the end of the thermometer and remove it from the patient's mouth.	___	___
12. Read the last colored dot on the thermometer and record the reading.	___	___
13. Discard the thermometer.	___	___

	Yes	No
14. Place the signal light within reach and check to make sure the patient is comfortable.	___	___
15. Unscreen the patient.	___	___
16. Wash your hands.	___	___
17. Report abnormal temperature readings to the nurse.	___	___

Procedure Completed ______________________ **Date** ______________________

Notes ____

____

____

PROCEDURE

OBRA SP

USING A DIGITAL THERMOMETER

Standard Precautions ☐ Handwashing ☐ Gloving ☐ Gowning ☐ Masking

Introductory Tasks ☐ Gather Equipment ☐ Identify/Introduce/Explain ☐ Provide Privacy

	Yes	No
6. Place a probe cover over the probe.	___	___
7. Ask the patient to wet his or her lips.	___	___
8. Insert the probe under the patient's tongue.	___	___
9. Hold the probe in place.	___	___
10. When the temperature measurement is complete, the probe will emit a tone, or, on some models, a light will flash or stay on continuously. When you hear or see the signal, gently grasp the end of the thermometer and remove it from the patient's mouth.	___	___
11. Read and record the patient's temperature.	___	___
12. Press the button that ejects the probe cover. Discard the cover into the wastebasket.	___	___
13. Place the probe back in the probe holder.	___	___
14. Place the signal light within reach and check to make sure the patient is comfortable.	___	___
16. Place the thermometer in the charging unit.	___	___
17. Unscreen the patient.	___	___
18. Wash your hands.	___	___
19. Report abnormal temperature readings to the nurse.	___	___
20. Record the measurement in the proper place.	___	___

Procedure Completed ______________________ **Date** ______________________

Notes ______________________

____

____

PROCEDURE

USING A STETHOSCOPE TO MEASURE AN APICAL PULSE

Standard Precautions ☐ Handwashing ☐ Gloving ☐ Gowning ☐ Masking

Introductory Tasks ☐ Gather Equipment ☐ Identify/Introduce/Explain ☐ Provide Privacy

	Yes	No
6. Using alcohol wipes, clean the diaphragm and earpieces of the stethoscope.	___	___
7. Hold the diaphragm in your hand to warm it before placing it on the patient's skin.	___	___
8. Position the earpieces in your ears.	___	___
9. Place the diaphragm directly over the artery. Keep the diaphragm in position by using the tips of your index and middle fingers.	___	___
10. Check to be sure the tubing that connects the diaphragm to the earpieces is free and clear of any objects.	___	___
11. When you are finished measuring, remove the stethoscope from the patient and then from your ears. Record your measurement.	___	___
12. Place the signal light within reach and check to make sure the patient is comfortable.	___	___
13. Wipe the earpieces and the diaphragm with alcohol wipes.	___	___
14. Store the stethoscope in its appropriate place.	___	___
15. Wash your hands.	___	___
16. Report and record the measurement in the proper place.	___	___

Procedure Completed ______________________ **Date** ______________________

Notes ______________________

____

____

PROCEDURE

OBRA SP

MEASURING A RADIAL PULSE

Standard Precautions	☐ Handwashing	☐ Gloving	☐ Gowning	☐ Masking
Introductory Tasks	☐ Gather Equipment	☐ Identify/Introduce/Explain	☐ Provide Privacy	

	Yes	**No**
6. Locate the radial pulse in the patient's wrist using your middle two or three fingers.	___	___
7. Note the strength and regularity of the pulse.	___	___
8. Begin counting the pulse beats and continue counting for one minute.	___	___
9. Record the pulse rate, force, and rhythm.	___	___
10. Place the signal light within reach and check to make sure the patient is comfortable.	___	___
11. Unscreen the patient.	___	___
12. Wash your hands.	___	___
13. Report readings to the nurse immediately if the patient's pulse rate is less than 60 beats per minute or greater than 100 beats per minute, or if any irregularities are heard. Bradycardia is a condition with less than 60 pulse beats per minute. Tachycardia is a condition with more than 100 beats per minute.	___	___

Procedure Completed ______________________ **Date** ______________

Notes ____

____

____

PROCEDURE

MEASURING AN APICAL-RADIAL PULSE

Standard Precautions ☐ Handwashing ☐ Gloving ☐ Gowning ☐ Masking

Introductory Tasks ☐ Gather Equipment ☐ Identify/Introduce/Explain ☐ Provide Privacy

	Yes	No
7. Remove or reach under the shirt or gown to expose the left nipple.	___	___
8. Wipe the earpieces of the stethoscope with alcohol wipes and place them in your ears.	___	___
9. Place the diaphragm in your hand to warm it.	___	___
10. Locate the apical pulse.	___	___
11. Ask your helper to locate the radial pulse.	___	___
12. Signal when you will begin counting.	___	___
13. Begin counting the pulse and continue for one minute.	___	___
14. After one minute, signal for the counting to stop.	___	___
15. Re-cover the patient's chest.	___	___
16. Record the apical and radial pulses. To obtain the pulse deficit, subtract the radial pulse from the apical pulse. Note the strength and regularity of the pulse.	___	___
17. Place the signal light within reach and check to make sure the patient is comfortable.	___	___
18. Unscreen the patient.	___	___
19. Wash your hands.	___	___
20. Report readings to the nurse immediately if the patient's apical pulse rate is less than 60 beats per minute or greater than 100 beats per minute, or if any irregularities are heard.	___	___
21. Record the measurement in the proper place.	___	___

Procedure Completed ______________________ **Date** ______________

Notes ____

____

____

PROCEDURE

OBRA SP

OBSERVING AND MEASURING A PATIENT'S RESPIRATION

Standard Precautions ☐ Handwashing ☐ Gloving ☐ Gowning ☐ Masking

Introductory Tasks ☐ Gather Equipment ☐ Identify/Introduce/Explain ☐ Provide Privacy

	Yes	No
6. Locate the radial pulse in the patient's wrist using your middle three fingers.	___	___
7. Note the strength and regularity of the pulse.	___	___
8. Begin counting the pulse beats and continue counting for 1 minute.	___	___
9. Keep your three fingers on the patient's wrist. Do not tell the patient that you are now going to measure respirations.	___	___
10. When you see the patient's chest rise, begin counting respirations. Each time the chest rises and falls, count one respiration. Continue counting for 1 minute.	___	___
11. While you are counting, observe the patient's breathing. Notice if the patient experiences any difficulty breathing. Check to see whether both sides of the chest rise and fall equally. Observe whether the breaths are regular, and whether they are deep or shallow. Listen for noises while the patient is breathing.	___	___
12. After 1 minute has elapsed, stop counting. This is the respiratory rate.	___	___
13. Record the respiratory rate and your observations of the patient's breathing.	___	___
14. Place the signal light within reach and check to make sure the patient is comfortable.	___	___
15. Wash your hands.	___	___
16. Report any abnormal reading to the nurse immediately, and record your measurement in the proper place.	___	___

Procedure Completed ______________________ **Date** ______________

Notes ____

____

____

PROCEDURE

OBRA SP

MEASURING A PATIENT'S BLOOD PRESSURE

Standard Precautions	☐ Handwashing	☐ Gloving	☐ Gowning	☐ Masking
Introductory Tasks	☐ Gather Equipment	☐ Identify/Introduce/Explain		☐ Provide Privacy

	Yes	No
6. Using alcohol wipes, clean the diaphragm and the earpieces of the stethoscope.	___	___
7. Ask the patient to sit or lie still.	___	___
8. Place the patient's arm in a position level with the heart, with the palm of the hand facing up.	___	___
9. Uncover the patient's arm.	___	___
10. Squeeze the cuff on the sphygmomanometer to make sure there is no air in the cuff. Close the valve on the bulb.	___	___
11. Locate the patient's brachial artery. Place the cuff on the patient's arm, at least 1 inch above the elbow, with the tube over the brachial artery. Make sure the cuff is evenly positioned around the arm and then tighten it so it fits snugly.	___	___
12. Put the stethoscope around your neck and insert the earpieces in your ears.	___	___
13. Find the patient's radial artery.	___	___
14. Explain to the patient that as the cuff inflates, he or she will feel a tightness in the arm that may be uncomfortable. Begin inflating the cuff by pumping the bulb with your other hand.	___	___
15. Notice when you can no longer feel the pulse. Inflate the cuff an additional 30 mm after you no longer feel the patient's pulse.	___	___
16. Place the diaphragm of the stethoscope over the patient's brachial artery.	___	___
17. Turn the valve on the sphygmomanometer counterclockwise and begin to evenly deflate the cuff at a rate of 2 to 4 mm per second.	___	___
18. Notice the reading on the scale when you first hear a sound. This is the patient's systolic reading.	___	___
19. As you continue to deflate the cuff, notice the reading on the scale when you no longer hear sound. This is the diastolic reading.	___	___
20. Continue letting air out of the cuff until it is completely deflated. Remove the cuff from the patient's arm. Remove the stethoscope.	___	___
21. Record the patient's blood pressure reading.	___	___
22. Clean the diaphragm and earpieces of the stethoscope with alcohol wipes.	___	___
23. Place the signal light within reach and check to make sure the patient is comfortable.	___	___
24. Unscreen the patient.	___	___
25. Place all equipment back where it belongs.	___	___

	Yes	No
26. Wash your hands.	___	___
27. Report abnormal blood pressure readings to the nurse.	___	___

Procedure Completed ______________________ **Date** ______________

Notes ____

____

____

PROCEDURE OBRA SP

MEASURING HEIGHT AND WEIGHT OF AN AMBULATORY PATIENT

Standard Precautions ☐ Handwashing ☐ Gloving ☐ Gowning ☐ Masking

Introductory Tasks ☐ Gather Equipment ☐ Identify/Introduce/Explain ☐ Provide Privacy

	Yes	No
6. Place a paper towel over the platform of the scale.	___	___
7. Raise the rod that is used to measure height.	___	___
8. Check to make sure the weights are set at zero and that the balance bar moves freely.	___	___
9. Ask the patient to remove his or her bathrobe and shoes or slippers. Assist if necessary.	___	___
10. Ask the patient to stand on the scale, with good posture and with the arms at the sides. Assist if necessary.	___	___
11. Slide the weights on the upper and lower bars to positions close to the patient's estimated weight.	___	___
12. When the balance pointer settles at a position halfway between the upper and lower bar guide, read the scale. To arrive at the patient's weight, add together the figures where the upper and lower weights are positioned. (For example, if the large weight is on 150 lbs. and the small weight is on 24 lbs., the patient's weight is 174 lbs.)	___	___
13. Record the patient's weight.	___	___
14. Ask the patient to stand very straight facing you.	___	___
15. Slide the movable point on the ruler down until it touches the top of the patient's head. This is the patient's height measurement.	___	___
16. Record the patient's height.	___	___
17. Help the patient step off the scale and put on the bathrobe and shoes or slippers. Assist the patient in returning to the chair or bed.	___	___
18. Place the signal light within reach and check to make sure the patient is comfortable.	___	___

	Yes	No
19. Remove and discard the paper covering the platform of the scale.	___	___
20. Wash your hands.	___	___

Procedure Completed ______________________ **Date** ______________________

Notes ______________________

____

____

PROCEDURE

OBRA SP

MEASURING HEIGHT AND WEIGHT OF A BEDRIDDEN PATIENT

Standard Precautions ☐ Handwashing ☐ Gloving ☐ Gowning ☐ Masking

Introductory Tasks ☐ Gather Equipment ☐ Identify/Introduce/Explain ☐ Provide Privacy

	Yes	No
6. Check to be sure the scale is in good condition (no areas of fraying, no straps that do not close properly).	___	___
7. Make sure the side rail on the far side of the bed is in the raised and locked position. Lower the side rail on the side of the bed near you.	___	___
8. Fanfold the top linens down to the foot of the bed.	___	___
9. Make sure the patient is lying on his or her back in good body alignment. The arms and legs should be straight. If the patient has contracted limbs, measure each segment (head to shoulder, upper back, lower back, and so on) separately.	___	___
10. Using the pencil, make a small mark on the bottom sheet at the top of the patients' head.	___	___
11. Make a small pencil mark on the sheet where the patient's feet end.	___	___
12. Anchor the tape measure at one end. With the tape measure, measure the distance between the two pencil marks. This is the patient's height.	___	___
13. Record the patient's height.	___	___
14. Remove the over-bed scale sling from its suspension straps. Position the sling under the patient as follows:	___	___

a. Ask the patient to turn on his or her side facing away from you. Assist if necessary.
b. Place the sling, folded lengthwise, under the patient.
c. Ask the patient to turn onto the side facing you. Assist if necessary. Raise the side rail on the side of the bed you have been working on.
d. Go to the other side of the bed and smooth out the sling under the patient.

	Yes	No
e. Ask the patient to resume lying flat on his or her back. f. Make sure the patient is positioned securely in the sling. g. Hook the sling to the suspension straps. Make sure the sling is securely attached.		
15. Move the lift frame into position over the bed. Lock the legs of the frame in the maximum open position.	___	___
16. Raise the head of the bed until the patient is in a sitting position.	___	___
17. Hook the suspension straps to the frame of the scale. Gently place the patient's arms inside the straps.	___	___
18. Slowly raise the sling until the patient's body is clear of the bed.	___	___
19. Slowly move the lift so that no part of the patient is making contact with the bed.	___	___
20. Move the weights on the scale until the scale is balanced.	___	___
21. Read and record the patient's weight.	___	___
22. Slowly move the sling back over the bed until it is centered.	___	___
23. Slowly release the sling, while guiding the patient back down toward the bed.	___	___
24. Reverse the procedure in Step 14 to remove the sling from underneath the patient.	___	___
25. Move the scale away from the bed.	___	___
26. Place the signal light within reach and check to make sure the patient is comfortable and in good body alignment.	___	___
27. Rearrange the top linens so that they cover the patient appropriately.	___	___
28. Raise and lock the side rail on the side of the bed where you have been working.	___	___
29. Unscreen the patient.	___	___
30. Return the over-bed scale to its storage area.	___	___
31. Wash your hands.	___	___
32. Report and record the measurements.	___	___

Procedure Completed ______________________________ **Date** ______________________

Notes ____

____

____

PROCEDURE

OBRA SP

WEIGHING A PATIENT IN A WHEELCHAIR

Step	Yes	No
1. If the wheelchair has not already been weighed, weigh the wheelchair: **a.** Take the wheelchair to the wheelchair scale. Balance the scale. **b.** Place the ramps of the chair on either side of the scale. **c.** Move the wheelchair onto the platform. Let go of the wheelchair. **d.** Record the wheelchair's weight.	___	___
2. Take the wheelchair to the patient's room.	___	___
3. Identify the patient, check the ID bracelet, and call the patient by name.	___	___
4. Introduce yourself.	___	___
5. Explain the procedure to the patient.	___	___
6. Wash your hands.	___	___
7. Provide privacy.	___	___
8. Make sure the bed wheels are locked. Make sure the wheelchair wheels are locked and the footrests are up.	___	___
9. Transfer the patient into the wheelchair.	___	___
10. Wheel the chair holding the patient to the wheelchair scale, with the wheelchair facing the ramp.	___	___
11. Push the wheelchair up the ramp onto the scale platform. Lock the wheels of the wheelchair.	___	___
12. Read and record the weight of the wheelchair and patient.	___	___
13. Unlock the wheels and gently pull the wheelchair down off the scale platform.	___	___
14. Wheel the patient back to his or her room. Return the patient to a chair or to bed.	___	___
15. Place the signal light within reach and check to make sure the patient is comfortable and in good body alignment.	___	___
16. To arrive at the patient's weight, subtract the weight of the wheelchair alone from the measurement of the wheelchair and patient together. Record the patient's weight.	___	___
17. Wash your hands.	___	___
18. Report and record the measurement.	___	___

Procedure Completed ______________________ **Date** ______________________

Notes ____

____

____

CHAPTER 21

NUTRITION

STUDY OBJECTIVES

Nutrition is necessary to sustain life. Patients receive nutrition in several ways. Special diets are used to improve or avoid problems associated with certain medical conditions. People often have specific cultural and religious dietary preferences.

- Patients receive nutrients from food and fluids by feeding themselves or being fed. They may also receive nutrition via intravenous therapy.
- Fluid balance is important to maintain good health. Too little fluid intake can cause dehydration. If fluid intake is greater than output, edema can result.
- Nursing assistants monitor intake by recording all food and fluid that the patient consumes. Fluid output is monitored by measuring urine.
- Patients should be fed slowly and in small amounts to avoid choking.
- Special diets can maintain or improve a medical condition.
- People who receive intravenous therapy are monitored for any changes near the infusion site, for leaks, level of fluid in the bag, and consistency of the drip.
- Some religions forbid the consumption of alcohol and caffeine. Others have strict rules about meat or dairy products.

KNOW YOUR TERMS

In the space provided, write the letter of the definition that best fits the numbered term.

__ 1. anorexia	a. An abnormal lack of bodily fluid.
__ 2. appetite	b. The delivery of medications, fluid, or nutrients through a needle inserted into a vein.
__ 3. carbohydrates	c. Swelling caused by excessive watery accumulation in tissues.
__ 4. dehydration	d. A container, usually of plastic or glass, marked with measurements.
__ 5. edema	e. Nutrients usable by the body for maintaining health and for growth.
— 6. emesis	f. Desire to eat.
__ 7. fat	g. A substance that is ingested into the body and provides the fuel for growth and maintaining health.
__ 8. graduate	h. A plant or animal substance needed to build and rebuild cells; a substance of the body that is an essential part of every cell.
__ 9. intravenous (IV) therapy	i. Any of various substances essential to the body in minute amounts.
__10. mineral	j. The act of vomiting.
__11. nutrient	k. Plant or animal compound made up of greasy, semisolid material; greasy tissue found in the human body.
__12. nutrition	l. An inorganic substance present in the body in minuscule amounts and essential to healthy body functioning.
__13. protein	m. A lack of appetite for food.
__14. vitamin	n. Nutrients, usually formed from green plants.

TEST YOUR KNOWLEDGE

Write the word(s) that best completes the statement.

1. ____________ is the process of taking food and fluids into the body for growth, healing, and maintaining body function.
2. The most important nutrient is ____________.
3. The body receives energy from the consumption of ____________.
4. A balanced diet includes foods from the ____________ different food groups.
5. ____________ occurs when the body does not take in as much fluid as it needs to function.

6. ______________ means "nothing by mouth."
7. A ______________ is a container for measuring fluids.
8. ______________ therapy is a way to receive nutrition.
9. ______________ is the desire for food.
10. ______________ is the loss of appetite.

THINK ABOUT THE ISSUES

1. How do you rate your own diet? List some ways you could improve your diet.
2. Food preferences are often based on a person's culture or religion. Sometimes food preferences may interfere with medically necessary special diets. Do you think a person should be forced to follow a special diet? Why or why not?

CHECK YOUR SKILLS

In the following procedure checklists, check each task box that applies and answer yes or no to each step you have completed. If possible, have your instructor sign off when you have completed a procedure.

PROCEDURE

OBRA SP

PREPARING A PATIENT FOR A MEAL

Standard Precautions ☐ Handwashing ☐ Gloving ☐ Gowning ☐ Masking

Introductory Tasks ☐ Gather Equipment ☐ Identify/Introduce/Explain ☐ Provide Privacy

	Yes	No
6. Assist the patient as necessary with oral hygiene.	___	___
7. Ask the patient if the bedpan or urinal is needed. If the patient is able to walk to the bathroom, offer the slippers and robe. Assist if necessary.	___	___
8. Provide the patient with the wash basin, soap, and a washcloth and towel for handwashing. Assist if necessary.	___	___
9. If the patient is able to sit in a chair for meals: **a.** Provide the robe and slippers. **b.** Help the patient to the chair. **c.** Place the over-bed table in a comfortable position for eating (waist level is usually best). Make sure it is clear of objects and the surface is clean. Go to Step 11.	___	___

	Yes	No
10. If the patient is unable to get out of bed to eat: a. If instructed, make sure the bed rails on both sides of the bed are in the raised and locked position. b. Raise the head of the bed until the patient is in a sitting position. c. Move the over-bed table to a comfortable position for eating. Make sure it is clear of objects and the surface is clean.	___	___
11. Make sure the patient can reach the signal light.	___	___
12. Unscreen the patient.	___	___
13. Wash your hands.	___	___

Procedure Completed ______________________ **Date** ______________________

Notes ____

____

____

PROCEDURE

OBRA SP

SERVING A MEAL TO A PATIENT OR RESIDENT WHO CANNOT GO TO THE DINING ROOM

Standard Precautions ☐ Handwashing ☐ Gloving ☐ Gowning ☐ Masking

Introductory Tasks ☐ Gather Equipment ☐ Identify/Introduce/Explain ☐ Provide Privacy

	Yes	No
4. Check to make sure the tray is the correct diet for the patient. Be sure it contains all the items noted on the dietary card.	___	___
5. Help the patient move to a sitting position in bed or in the chair.	___	___
6. Place the over-bed table in a comfortable position for eating. Make sure it is clear of objects and the surface is clean.	___	___
7. Uncover food that is covered. Open all cartons, boxes, and containers. If there is any food the patient cannot cut on his or her own, provide assistance.	___	___
8. Make sure the patient can reach the utensils, napkin, and all food.	___	___
9. If the patient does not need further assistance, leave the room.	___	___
10. When the patient is finished eating, return to the room and remove the tray. If ordered, measure and record what foods were eaten and the quantities of each.	___	___
11. If any food or drink was spilled, clean it up now.	___	___
12. If appropriate, help the patient return to bed.	___	___

	Yes	No
13. Assist with oral hygiene as needed.	___	___
14. Check to make sure the patient is comfortable and that the body is aligned properly.	___	___
15. Make sure the signal light is within the patient's reach.	___	___
16. Wash your hands.	___	___

Procedure Completed ______________________ **Date** ______________

Notes ____

____

____

PROCEDURE

OBRA SP

SERVING A MEAL TO A BLIND PATIENT

Standard Precautions ☐ Handwashing ☐ Gloving ☐ Gowning ☐ Masking

Introductory Tasks ☐ Gather Equipment ☐ Identify/Introduce/Explain ☐ Provide Privacy

	Yes	No
5. Help the patient move to a sitting position.	___	___
6. Place the over-bed table in a comfortable position for you and the patient. Make sure it is clear of objects and the surface is clean.	___	___
7. Check to make sure the food tray is the correct diet for the patient. Be sure it contains all the items noted on the dietary card.	___	___
8. Place a napkin under the patient's chin.	___	___
9. Remove the covers from all food that is covered. Open all cartons, boxes, and containers. Place a straw in the cold beverage container. Prepare the food into small servings that will take up half a spoonful at most. Cut all food that is not bite-sized. Butter breads, season foods, and fix coffee or tea according to the patient's preferences and in accordance with any dietary restrictions. As you are doing these things, describe the food on the tray.	___	___
10. Ask the patient to imagine that the tray is a clock face. Use the numbers on a clock to describe the food's position to the patient. For example, the bread is at 9 o'clock.	___	___
11. If possible, encourage the patient to feed him- or herself. Tell the patient the position of the spoon. Guide the patient's hand to the spoon if necessary. Go to Step 16.	___	___

	Yes	No
12. If the patient cannot feed him- or herself, follow Steps 13 through 15.	___	___
13. Feed the patient the food on the tray in a logical order (appetizer, then the main course, followed by coffee or tea and dessert). If the appetizer is soup or juice, you can alternate either of those with the main course since liquids, such as soup or juice, may fill the patient up too fast. It is better for the patient to have at least some of each item on the tray. Fill the spoon half full with food. As you bring the spoon to the patient's mouth, tell the patient what it is. Warn the patient if the food is hot. Make sure it is not too hot to be served. (To test the heat of the food, let one drop of it fall onto your finger and feel the temperature before serving. Never touch food that is then going to be served to the patient.)	___	___
14. Place the tip of the spoon in one side of the patient's mouth. Remove the spoon once the patient has taken the food off the spoon. Wait until the patient has finished chewing before offering something to drink. Do not rush the patient.	___	___
15. Offer the patient drinks between spoonfuls of solid food. To serve liquids, guide the straw (if a cold beverage) or the edge of the cup (if a hot beverage) to the patient's lips.	___	___
16. When the patient finishes, help him or her wipe the mouth with a clean napkin.	___	___
17. Remove the tray and the over-bed table. If ordered, measure and record what foods were eaten and the quantities of each.	___	___
18. If any food or drink was spilled, clean it up now.	___	___
19. Check to make sure that the patient is comfortable and the body is aligned properly.	___	___
20. Make sure the signal light is within the patient's reach.	___	___
21. Wash your hands.	___	___

Procedure Completed ______________________ **Date** ______________________

Notes ____

____

____

PROCEDURE

OBRA SP

FEEDING A PATIENT WHO CANNOT FEED HIMSELF OR HERSELF

Standard Precautions ☐ Handwashing ☐ Gloving ☐ Gowning ☐ Masking

Introductory Tasks ☐ Gather Equipment ☐ Identify/Introduce/Explain ☐ Provide Privacy

	Yes	No
5. Help the patient move to a sitting position.	___	___
6. Place the over-bed table in a comfortable position for you and the patient. Make sure it is clear of objects and the surface is clean.	___	___
7. Check to make sure the food tray is the correct diet for the patient. Be sure it contains all the items noted on the dietary card.	___	___
8. Place a napkin under the patient's chin.	___	___
9. Remove the covers from all food that is covered. Open all cartons, boxes, and containers. Place a straw in the cold beverage container. Prepare the food into small servings that will take up half a spoonful at most. Cut all food that is not bite-sized. Butter breads, season foods, and fix coffee or tea according to the patient's preferences and in accordance with any dietary restrictions.	___	___
10. Feed the patient the food on the tray in a logical order (appetizer, such as soup or juice, then the main course, followed by coffee or tea and dessert). Fill the spoon half full with food. Warn the patient if the food is hot. Make sure it is not too hot to be served.	___	___
11. Place the tip of the spoon in one side of the patient's mouth. Remove the spoon once the patient has taken the food off the spoon. Wait until the patient finishes chewing before offering something to drink. Do not rush the patient.	___	___
12. Offer the patient drinks between spoonfuls of solid food. To serve liquids, guide the straw (if a cold beverage) or the edge of the cup (if a hot beverage) to the patient's lips.	___	___
13. When the patient finishes, wipe the mouth with a clean napkin.	___	___
14. Remove the tray and the over-bed table. If ordered, measure and record the type of food eaten and the quantity consumed.	___	___
15. If any food or drink was spilled, clean it up now.	___	___
16. Check to make sure the patient is comfortable and that the body is aligned properly.	___	___
17. Make sure the signal light is within the patient's reach.	___	___
18. Wash your hands.	___	___

Procedure Completed ____________________ **Date** ____________________

Notes ____

____

____

PROCEDURE

SERVING NUTRIENTS (SNACKS) BETWEEN MEALS

Standard Precautions ☐ Handwashing ☐ Gloving ☐ Gowning ☐ Masking

Introductory Tasks ☐ Gather Equipment ☐ Identify/Introduce/Explain ☐ Provide Privacy

	Yes	No
4. Help the patient move to a sitting position. Raise the head of the bed.	___	___
5. Wash the patient's hands.	___	___
6. Prepare the food for the patient. Open cartons and containers.	___	___
7. Offer the food to the patient. Provide assistance if the patient requires it.	___	___
8. When the patient finishes, remove the tray and wash the patient's hands.	___	___
9. If ordered, measure and record the type of food eaten and the quantity consumed.	___	___
10. If any food or drink was spilled, clean it up now.	___	___
11. Lower the bed to a comfortable position for the patient.	___	___
12. Check to make sure the patient is in good body alignment.	___	___
13. Make sure the signal light is within the patient's reach.	___	___
14. Wash your hands.	___	___

Procedure Completed ______________________ **Date** ______________________

Notes ____

____

____

PROCEDURE

OBRA SP

MEASURING AND RECORDING THE INTAKE OF NUTRITION

Standard Precautions ☐ Handwashing ☐ Gloving ☐ Gowning ☐ Masking

Introductory Tasks ☐ Gather Equipment ☐ Identify/Introduce/Explain ☐ Provide Privacy

	Yes	No
4. Pour the liquid that is left over from the patient's serving into the graduate.	___	___
5. Place the graduate on a level surface. At eye level, read the measurement of the amount of liquid.	___	___
6. Determine the full amount of the serving (usually listed on the I & O record).	___	___
7. Subtract the leftover amount from the full serving amount (for example, 300 mL full serving - 140 mL left = 160 mL consumed).	___	___
8. Note this amount.	___	___
9. Empty the graduate.	___	___
10. Repeat Steps 4 through 10 for all other leftover liquids. Make sure the graduate is empty before pouring another liquid into the container.	___	___
11. Add the amounts noted in Steps 9 and 11. This is the total intake.	___	___
12. Record the time and the amount as instructed.	___	___
13. Clean all the equipment and return it to its proper storage place.	___	___
14. Wash your hands.	___	___

Procedure Completed ______________________ **Date** ______________

Notes ____

____

____

PROCEDURE

SUPPLYING DRINKING WATER TO ABLE PATIENTS

Standard Precautions ☐ Handwashing ☐ Gloving ☐ Gowning ☐ Masking

Introductory Tasks ☐ Gather Equipment ☐ Identify/Introduce/Explain ☐ Provide Privacy

Step	Yes	No
2. Ask the nurse for a list of patients who have special fluid orders.	___	___
3. Place paper towels on the top shelf of the cart. Arrange the equipment on the cart in a way that makes it easy for you to distribute the water.	___	___
4. Push the cart until you are just outside the patient's room. Identify the patient(s) in the room. Check the ID bracelet.	___	___
5. Check the list of patients with special fluid orders.	___	___
6. Locate the empty water pitcher. If any water remains in the pitcher, empty it into the bathroom sink.	___	___
7. Using water from the bathroom tap or from the large pitcher on the cart, fill the patient's pitcher half full with water.	___	___
8. If the patient is allowed to have ice, scoop some ice from the ice chest into the pitcher.	___	___
9. Position the pitcher on the over-bed table. Place a clean disposable cup and straw next to the pitcher.	___	___
10. Pour water into the disposable cup. Make sure the patient can reach the cup, straw, and pitcher.	___	___
11. Take the cart to the next room. Repeat Steps 4 through 10 for each patient.	___	___
12. When you finish, empty the ice chest and pitcher. Wash all equipment before returning it to its storage area.	___	___
13. Wash your hands.	___	___

Procedure Completed ______________________ **Date** ______________

Notes ____

____

____

PROCEDURE

GIVING DRINKING WATER TO PATIENTS WHO NEED ASSISTANCE

Standard Precautions ☐ Handwashing ☐ Gloving ☐ Gowning ☐ Masking

Introductory Tasks ☐ Gather Equipment ☐ Identify/Introduce/Explain ☐ Provide Privacy

	Yes	No
2. Ask the nurse for a list of patients who have special fluid orders.	___	___
3. Place paper towels on the top shelf of the cart. Arrange the equipment on the cart in a way that makes it easy for you to distribute water to patients.	___	___
4. Push the cart to a patient's room. Identify the patient(s) in the room. Check the ID bracelet.	___	___
5. Check the list of patients with special fluid orders.	___	___
6. Locate the empty water pitcher. If any water remains in the pitcher, empty it into the bathroom sink.	___	___
7. Using water from the bathroom tap or from the large pitcher on the cart, fill the patient's pitcher half-full with water.	___	___
8. If the patient is allowed to have ice, scoop some ice from the ice chest into the pitcher.	___	___
9. Position the pitcher on the over-bed table. Place a clean disposable cup and straw next to the pitcher.	___	___
10. Pour water into the disposable cup.	___	___
11. Offer the patient a drink. If the patient wants a drink, guide the straw to the patient's lips.	___	___
12. When the patient is finished, wipe the mouth with a clean napkin.	___	___
13. Take the cart to the next room. Repeat Steps 4 through 12 for each patient who needs assistance drinking.	___	___
14. When you finish, empty the ice chest and pitcher. Wash all equipment before returning it to its storage area.	___	___
15. Wash your hands.	___	___

Procedure Completed ______________________________ **Date** ____________________

Notes ____

____

____

PROCEDURE

DRESSING A RESIDENT WHO HAS AN IV

Standard Precautions ☐ Handwashing ☐ Gloving ☐ Gowning ☐ Masking

Introductory Tasks ☐ Gather Equipment ☐ Identify/Introduce/Explain ☐ Provide Privacy

	Yes	No
5. Remove the gown or article of clothing from the arm without the IV.	___	___
6. Move the gown or item of clothing down the arm that has the IV. Slowly remove the arm and hand from the sleeve.	___	___
7. Keep the sleeve gathered. Slide your hand along the tubing to the IV solution container (the bag or bottle).	___	___
8. Remove the container from the pole. Slide the container and tubing over it. Hold the container above the resident's arm, and do not pull or tug on the tubing.	___	___
9. Replace the container on the pole.	___	___
10. Gather the sleeve of the clean gown that will go on the arm with the IV. Remove the container from the pole, and slip the sleeve over the bottle. Hang the container back on the pole.	___	___
11. Slide the sleeve over the tubing, hand, arm, and IV location. Then slide the sleeve onto the resident's shoulder.	___	___
12. Put the other side of the garment on the resident and fasten it.	___	___
13. Make sure the resident is comfortable.	___	___
14. Unscreen the resident, if appropriate, and remove the soiled garment.	___	___
15. Wash your hands.	___	___
16. Check the patient and the IV site.	___	___
17. Ask the nurse to check the IV flow rate.	___	___

Procedure Completed ______________________ **Date** ______________

Notes ____

____

____

PROCEDURE

ASSISTING THE RESIDENT WITH AN IV THERAPY CONNECTION TO WALK

	Yes	No
1. Identify the resident, introduce yourself, and explain the procedure.	___	___
2. Wash your hands.	___	___
3. Correctly position the portable IV pole before helping the resident walk.	___	___
4. Protect the position of the IV solution container, tubing, and needle. Allow slack in the tubing so the needle does not become dislodged.	___	___
5. If the position of the clamp appears to have changed, ask the nurse to check the IV flow rate.	___	___
6. If blood appears in the tubing, alert your supervisor.	___	___

Procedure Completed ______________________ **Date** ______________________

Notes ____

____

____

CHAPTER 22

Elimination and Sample Collections

Study Objectives

Elimination is an important natural life process. Nursing assistants perform many procedures that aid in or clean up after elimination. Urine, stool, and sputum testing is useful in making diagnoses of certain illnesses. Incontinence can be a frightening prospect for some patients. Helping patients maintain their dignity is an important part of personal care.

- Assisting ambulatory patients to the toilet includes helping them out of bed, making sure they wear slippers and a robe, escorting them to the toilet, and helping them clean themselves, if necessary.
- A portable commode is brought next to the bed and the patient is helped onto it. After elimination, the nursing assistants helps with any cleaning and cleans the commode.
- Offer the urinal to males at regular intervals. Help them sit or stand, if possible. Empty and clean the urinal after use.
- Patients who are bedridden need to use bedpans. Help the patient onto the bedpan, provide privacy, provide perineal care when the patient is finished, and clean the bedpan.
- Some incontinent patients can be trained to regain bladder and bowel control. If not, keep the patient as clean as possible.
- A catheter is a tube used to drain fluid from a body opening, especially urine from the bladder. Catheter care includes emptying the drainage bag, providing perineal care, and cleaning the catheter.
- A catheter empties liquid into a drainage bag where it can be observed, measured, and emptied.
- Urine samples are collected and tested for certain conditions. The patient may provide the urine sample in a cup, or the nursing assistant may take a sample.
- To check urine for the presence of stones, urine is strained through a paper or gauze strainer.
- Rectal tubes are used to relieve gas. Suppositories are used to soften stools that cause constipation. Both are inserted into the rectum.

- Stool samples are usually collected from a bedpan or specipan. They are then placed in a container for testing.
- Enemas are liquid solutions placed into the rectum to loosen stools and remove feces. An enema should always be given next to a bedpan or toileting facility.
- Colostomy and ileostomy appliances require emptying and cleaning as often as necessary. Deodorants are placed in the cleaned bag. Special powder is used to maintain the skin around the colostomy site.
- To collect a sputum sample, the patient is asked to cough up the sputum from the lungs into a cup.

KNOW YOUR TERMS

MATCHING EXERCISE I

In the space provided, write the letter of the definition that best fits the numbered term.

__ 1. abdominal distension	a. A metal or plastic device used by patients who are bedridden to urinate or defecate.
__ 2. Acetest	b. Infrequent or difficult passage of feces.
__ 3. bedpan	c. Gas in the stomach or intestines.
__ 4. cleansing enema	d. A rubber sheath placed over the penis and connected to tubing through which urine drains into a drainage bag.
__ 5. Clinitest	e. An enema that is prepackaged in a plastic bottle discarded after use.
__ 6. colostomy	f. The discharge of feces from the anus.
__ 7. commercial enema	g. A liquid solution placed into the rectum to loosen stools and remove feces.
__ 8. condom catheter	h. An inflammation of the bladder.
__ 9. constipation	i. The excretion of waste material from the body.
__10. cystitis	j. The waste discharged through the anus.
__11. defecation	k. Another name for a condom catheter.
__12. elimination	l. A commercial test for acetones and ketones in the urine, performed by adding a drop of urine to the Acetest tablet.
__13. enema	m. An artificial opening in the abdominal wall through which feces are passed.
__14. external urinary drainage (EUD) catheter	n. Abnormal swelling of the abdomen.
__15. feces	o. Another name for an indwelling catheter.
__16. flatulence	p. An artificial opening between the small intestine and the abdominal wall through which liquid feces pass.

__17. Foley catheter	q. A commercial test that measures the amount of glucose in a patient's urine in a solution that changes color.
__18. fracture pan	r. A bedpan specifically designed for use by patients with fractures.
__19. ileostomy	s. An enema that cleanses the lower intestines.

MATCHING EXERCISE II

__ 1. incontinence	a. Blood from a concealed or not visible hemorrhage.
__ 2. indwelling catheter	b. The opening in a colostomy.
__ 3. Keto-Diastix	c. Inability to control elimination.
__ 4. occult blood	d. Another name for a condom catheter.
__ 5. oil-retention enema	e. The surgical creation of an artificial opening in the body.
__ 6. ostomy	f. A type of enema that encourages the softening of constipated stool and subsequent defecation.
__ 7. rectal tube	g. A commercial test that uses a plastic strip to determine if glucose and ketones are in the urine.
__ 8. retention catheter	h. The act of discharging urine from the body.
__ 9. specipan	i. A catheter with a balloon at its tip that is inflated once it is inserted into the bladder.
__10. sputum	j. A tube inserted in the rectum to relieve flatulence or gas.
__11. stoma	k. A bullet-shaped waxy material inserted into the rectum to soften stools and ease constipation.
__12. stool	l. A vessel for urination.
__13. suppository	m. Expectorated matter.
__14. Testape	n. Feces.
__15. Texas catheter	o. A commercial test for glucose in urine performed by dipping a strip into the urine and checking the color change.
__16. urinal	p. Waste material secreted through the urinary tract.
__17. urination	q. Another name for an indwelling catheter.
__18. urine	r. A receptacle that fits under a toilet seat to collect urine and stool specimens.

TEST YOUR KNOWLEDGE

Write the word(s) that best completes the statement.

1. _____________ is the discharge of waste from the body.
2. Defecation is the discharge of _____________ from the body.
3. _____________ is the inability to control the passing of waste from the body.
4. Difficulty in fecal elimination is called _____________.
5. The excessive creation and buildup of gas in the stomach and intestines is called _____________.
6. Patients who are bedridden use a _____________ for elimination.
7. A _____________ is a tube used to drain fluid from the body.
8. A _____________-_____________ urine sample is collected after the perineal area is thoroughly cleaned.
9. The urine of patients with diabetes is tested for _____________ and _____________.
10. An _____________ is a liquid solution placed into the rectum to loosen stools and to remove feces.

THINK ABOUT THE ISSUES

1. Try to imagine needing help with elimination. How do you think you would feel?
2. List some of the ways you can help keep residents clean while still maintaining their dignity.

CHECK YOUR SKILLS

In the following procedure checklists, check each task box that applies and answer yes or no to each step you have completed. If possible, have your instructor sign off when you have completed a procedure.

PROCEDURE

ASSISTING A PATIENT WITH A PORTABLE COMMODE

Standard Precautions ☐ Handwashing ☐ Gloving ☐ Gowning ☐ Masking

Introductory Tasks ☐ Gather Equipment ☐ Identify/Introduce/Explain ☐ Provide Privacy

Step	Yes	No
5. Bring the commode close to the patient's bed. Remove the lid of the commode.	___	___
6. Help the patient sit on the side of the bed.	___	___
7. Assist the patient in putting on a robe and slippers.	___	___
8. Assist the patient to the commode. Make sure he or she is correctly positioned.	___	___
9. Cover the patient with the blanket.	___	___
10. Place the toilet paper and signal cord within reach. Tell the patient to signal when he or she is finished.	___	___
11. Wash your hands.	___	___
12. Leave the room and close the door.	___	___
13. Answer the signal immediately. Knock and pause before entering the room.	___	___
14. Wash your hands.	___	___
15. Put on your gloves.	___	___
16. Help the patient with perineal care. Make sure the patient is clean.	___	___
17. Remove your gloves.	___	___
18. Wash your hands.	___	___
19. Help the patient back into the bed or chair.	___	___
20. Make the patient comfortable and place the call signal within reach.	___	___
21. Put on a clean pair of gloves.	___	___
22. Cover and remove the container from the commode.	___	___
23. Take the container to the bathroom. Check urine or feces for color, odor, amount, and character. Measure the urine, if instructed. Collect a specimen if one has been ordered. Empty any remaining contents into the toilet.	___	___
24. Clean and disinfect the container.	___	___
25. Place the container back in the commode. Clean the commode, if necessary.	___	___
26. Remove your gloves.	___	___
27. Return supplies to their proper place for the next use.	___	___
28. Help the patient wash his or her hands using the wash basin, soap, and towel.	___	___
29. Unscreen the patient.	___	___

	Yes	No
30. Place dirty linens in the hamper.	___	___
31. Wash your hands.	___	___
32. Report your observations to the nurse.	___	___

Procedure Completed ______________________ **Date** ______________________

Notes ____

____

____

PROCEDURE

OBRA SP

GIVING A BEDPAN TO A PATIENT

Standard Precautions ☐ Handwashing ☐ Gloving ☐ Gowning ☐ Masking

Introductory Tasks ☐ Gather Equipment ☐ Identify/Introduce/Explain ☐ Provide Privacy

	Yes	No
5. Raise the bed to a comfortable working level. Raise the patient's head if this is permitted. The closer the patient is to a sitting position, the easier it is to use the bedpan.	___	___
6. Warm the bedpan, if necessary, by running warm water over it and drying it.	___	___
7. Lower the side rail, if applicable.	___	___
8. Position the patient so he or she is lying on the back, with the head elevated.	___	___
9. Fold the patient's gown up and out of the way.	___	___
10. Lower the bed linens, keeping the patient's lower body covered.	___	___
11. Ask the patient to flex the knees and raise the buttocks. You may need to slide your hand under the patient's back to help raise the buttocks.	___	___
12. Slide the bedpan under the patient. Make sure it is correctly placed.	___	___
13. If the patient is unable to help in getting on the bedpan, you can turn the patient away from you. Lower the head of the bed. Place the bedpan against the patient's buttocks, and push the bedpan down toward the patient. While securely holding the bedpan, roll the patient on his or her back. Raise the head of the bed.	___	___
14. Cover the patient.	___	___
15. Raise the side rail, if applicable.	___	___

	Yes	No
16. Place the toilet paper and signal cord within reach.	___	___
17. Instruct the patient to signal as soon as he or she is finished.	___	___
18. Wash your hands.	___	___
19. Leave the room.	___	___
20. Return as soon as the patient signals. Knock before you enter the room.	___	___
21. Wash your hands and put on gloves.	___	___
22. Lower the side rail, if applicable.	___	___
23. Ask the patient to raise the buttocks. Slide the bedpan out.	___	___
24. Cover the bedpan with the cover or a towel.	___	___
25. Help the patient with perineal care.	___	___
26. Raise the side rail, if applicable.	___	___
27. Take the bedpan to the bathroom. Measure the urine if instructed. Note the color, odor, amount, and character of urine or feces.	___	___
28. Empty the contents of the bedpan into the toilet.	___	___
29. Rinse the bedpan with cool water and then clean it with a disinfectant.	___	___
30. Remove the gloves.	___	___
31. Return the bedpan to the patient's bedside table.	___	___
32. Help the patient wash his or her hands.	___	___
33. Make the patient comfortable and place the signal cord within reach.	___	___
34. Unscreen the patient.	___	___
35. Wash your hands.	___	___
36. Report your observations to the nurse.	___	___

Procedure Completed ______________________________ **Date** ______________________

Notes ____

____

____

PROCEDURE

GIVING A FRACTURE PAN TO A PATIENT

Standard Precautions ☐ Handwashing ☐ Gloving ☐ Gowning ☐ Masking

Introductory Tasks ☐ Gather Equipment ☐ Identify/Introduce/Explain ☐ Provide Privacy

Step	Yes	No
5. Raise the bed to a comfortable working level. Raise the patient's head if this is permitted. The closer the patient is to a sitting position, the easier it is to use the fracture pan.	___	___
6. Warm the fracture pan, if necessary, by running warm water over it and drying it.	___	___
7. Lower the side rail, if applicable.	___	___
8. Position the patient on his or her back, with the head elevated.	___	___
9. Fold the patient's gown up and out of the way.	___	___
10. Lower the bed linens, keeping the patient's lower body covered.	___	___
11. Ask the patient to raise the buttocks. You may need to slide your hand under the patient's back to help raise the buttocks.	___	___
12. Slide the fracture pan under the patient. The smaller end goes under the buttocks. Make sure it is correctly placed.	___	___
13. If the patient is unable to get on the fracture pan, lower the head of the bed. Raise the buttocks with one arm and slide the fracture pan under the patient with the other arm.	___	___
14. Cover the patient.	___	___
15. Raise the side rail, if applicable.	___	___
16. Place the toilet paper and signal cord within reach.	___	___
17. Instruct the patient to signal as soon as he or she is finished. Tell patients whose intake/output is being measured not to place toilet paper in the pan.	___	___
18. Wash your hands.	___	___
19. Leave the room.	___	___
20. Return to the room as soon as the patient signals. Knock before you enter.	___	___
21. Put on gloves.	___	___
22. Lower the side rail, if applicable.	___	___
23. Slide the fracture pan out from under the patient.	___	___
24. Cover the pan with the cover or a towel.	___	___
25. Help with perineal care.	___	___
26. Raise the side rail, if applicable.	___	___

	Yes	No
27. Take the fracture pan to the bathroom. Measure the urine, if instructed. Note the color, odor, amount, and character of urine or feces.	___	___
28. Empty the contents of the fracture pan into the toilet.	___	___
29. Rinse the pan in cool water and then clean it with a disinfectant.	___	___
30. Remove your gloves.	___	___
31. Return the fracture pan to the patient's bedside table.	___	___
32. Help the patient wash his or her hands.	___	___
33. Make the patient comfortable and place the signal cord within reach.	___	___
34. Unscreen the patient.	___	___
35. Wash your hands.	___	___
36. Report your observations to the nurse.	___	___

Procedure Completed ______________________ **Date** ______________________

Notes ____

____

____

PROCEDURE

OBRA

SP

OFFERING A URINAL TO A MALE PATIENT

Standard Precautions ☐ Handwashing ☐ Gloving ☐ Gowning ☐ Masking

Introductory Tasks ☐ Gather Equipment ☐ Identify/Introduce/Explain ☐ Provide Privacy

	Yes	No
5. Help the patient to a standing position if the patient is able.	___	___
6. If the patient cannot stand, help him to lie on his back, with the bed raised at a 45° angle.	___	___
7. If the patient is lying down, pull back the linens.	___	___
8. Place the flat side of the urinal down on the mattress. Instruct the patient to place his penis into the urinal opening and urinate normally. If he cannot do this himself, you should help him. Wear gloves if you need to assist.	___	___
9. Cover the patient with the linens and place the signal cord within reach.	___	___
10. Wash your hands.	___	___
11. Leave the room and close the door.	___	___

	Yes	No
12. Answer the signal immediately. Knock and pause before entering the room.	___	___
13. Put on your gloves.	___	___
14. Remove the urinal.	___	___
15. Make the patient comfortable and place the signal cord within reach.	___	___
16. Take the urinal into the bathroom. Observe the urine for color, odor, amount, and character.	___	___
17. Measure the urine, if instructed. Collect a specimen if one has been ordered.	___	___
18. Empty the contents of the urinal into the toilet.	___	___
19. Rinse the urinal with cool water, then clean and disinfect it.	___	___
20. Replace the urinal in the patient's bedside stand or hang it on the resident's bed within reach.	___	___
21. Remove your gloves.	___	___
22. Help the patient wash his hands using the wash basin, soap, and towel.	___	___
23. Wash your hands.	___	___
24. Make the patient comfortable and place the signal cord within reach.	___	___
25. Report your observations to the nurse.	___	___

Procedure Completed ______________________ **Date** ______________________

Notes ____

____

____

PROCEDURE

OBRA SP

CARING FOR A CATHETER

Standard Precautions ☐ Handwashing ☐ Gloving ☐ Gowning ☐ Masking

Introductory Tasks ☐ Gather Equipment ☐ Identify/Introduce/Explain ☐ Provide Privacy

	Yes	No
5. Raise the bed to a comfortable working position.	___	___
6. Lower the side rail, if applicable.	___	___
7. Cover the patient with the bath blanket; then fanfold the top linens to the foot of the bed so you do not expose the patient.	___	___
8. Place the bed protector under the patient's buttocks.	___	___

	Yes	No
9. Put on your gloves.	___	___
10. Perform perineal care.	___	___
11. Open the catheter care kit (if used by your facility). Otherwise, use a washcloth.	___	___
12. Apply solution to the applicators or washcloths.	___	___
13. For female patients: Separate the labia. Check for crusts or abnormal drainage. Use the applicator to swab solution on the labia. Wipe from front to back. Use each applicator for only one swab. Throw the applicator in the biohazard waste bag after use.	___	___
14. For male patients: Retract the foreskin of an uncircumcised male. Check for crusts or abnormal drainage. Use the applicator to swab solution on the head of the penis. Use each applicator for only one swab. Throw the applicator in the biohazard waste bag after use.	___	___
15. Clean the catheter, starting at the urinary meatus and working down about 4 inches toward the drainage bag connection. Clean in a circular motion around the catheter as you work down. Hold the catheter in place as you clean it. Use each applicator for just one wipe. Avoid pulling on the catheter.	___	___
16. Make sure the catheter is taped properly and the tubing is secure.	___	___
17. Remove the bed protector.	___	___
18. Remove your gloves and wash your hands.	___	___
19. Cover the patient with the bed linens and slip the bath blanket out.	___	___
20. Make the patient comfortable and place the signal cord within reach.	___	___
21. Unscreen the patient.	___	___
22. Discard the dirty linens.	___	___
23. Clean all the equipment and store it for the next use.	___	___
24. Report your observations to the nurse.	___	___

Procedure Completed ______________________________ **Date** ______________________

Notes ____

____

____

PROCEDURE

APPLYING A CONDOM CATHETER TO A MALE PATIENT

Standard Precautions ☐ Handwashing ☐ Gloving ☐ Gowning ☐ Masking

Introductory Tasks ☐ Gather Equipment ☐ Identify/Introduce/Explain ☐ Provide Privacy

	Yes	No
5. Raise the bed to a good working position.	___	___
6. Lower the side rail, if applicable.	___	___
7. Cover the patient with a bath blanket; then fanfold the top linens down to the foot of the bed so you do not expose the patient.	___	___
8. Place the bed protector under the buttocks.	___	___
9. Put on your gloves.	___	___
10. Secure the drainage bag to the bed frame, or have the leg bag ready. Make sure the drain is closed. If the patient is already wearing a condom catheter, perform Steps 11-14.	___	___
11. Remove the tape or apply a skin prep adhesive remover and roll the condom toward the head of the penis.	___	___
12. Disconnect the drainage tube. Keep the top of the drainage tube clean by placing it in an aseptic container.	___	___
13. Discard the tape and condom in the waste bag.	___	___
14. Perform perineal care.	___	___
15. Remove the backing from the new condom.	___	___
16. Hold the patient's penis and roll the condom over the penis.	___	___
17. Leave a 1-inch space between the end of the penis and the catheter.	___	___
18. Use the tape to secure the condom on the penis. Apply tape in a spiral so the ends of the tape do not meet. If using a skin prep adhesive, apply it over the condom instead of the tape.	___	___
19. Connect the condom to the tubing.	___	___
20. Coil the extra tubing on the bed or attach it to the leg bag.	___	___
21. Remove the bed protector.	___	___
22. Cover the patient with the bed linens and slip out the bath blanket.	___	___
23. Make the patient comfortable and place the signal cord within reach.	___	___
24. Unscreen the patient.	___	___
25. Open the drainage bag and empty it into the graduate.	___	___
26. If instructed, measure and record the amount of urine before emptying it in the toilet.	___	___

	Yes	No
27. Discard the waste bag.	___	___
28. Discard the dirty linens.	___	___
29. Clean all equipment and store it for the next use.	___	___
30. Remove your gloves.	___	___
31. Wash your hands.	___	___
32. Report your observations to the nurse.	___	___

Procedure Completed ______________________________ **Date** ____________________

Notes ____

____

____

PROCEDURE

OBRA SP

EMPTYING A URINE DRAINAGE BAG AND MEASURING URINARY OUTPUT

Standard Precautions ☐ Handwashing ☐ Gloving ☐ Gowning ☐ Masking

Introductory Tasks ☐ Gather Equipment ☐ Identify/Introduce/Explain ☐ Provide Privacy

	Yes	No
6. Place a paper towel on the floor and place the graduate under the drain of the drainage bag on the paper towel.	___	___
7. Open the drain and let the urine run into the graduate, without touching the sides of the graduate.	___	___
8. Close the drain. Wipe it with the alcohol swab.	___	___
9. Replace the drain in the holder.	___	___
10. Make the patient comfortable and place the signal cord within reach.	___	___
11. Unscreen the patient.	___	___
12. Measure the urinary output by placing the graduate on a level surface at eye level. Note the amount and character of the urine.	___	___
13. Record the amount of urine.	___	___
14. Wash and dry the graduate and store it for the next use.	___	___
15. Remove and dispose of your gloves.	___	___

	Yes	No
16. Wash your hands.	___	___
17. Report the amount of urine collected and your observations to the nurse.	___	___

Procedure Completed ______________________ **Date** ______________________

Notes ____

____

____

PROCEDURE

COLLECTING A ROUTINE URINE SAMPLE

Standard Precautions ☐ Handwashing ☐ Gloving ☐ Gowning ☐ Masking

Introductory Tasks ☐ Gather Equipment ☐ Identify/Introduce/Explain ☐ Provide Privacy

	Yes	No
6. Ask the patient to urinate in the bedpan, urinal, or specipan. If the patient is able, he or she can go to the bathroom to urinate and provide a sample in the specimen container.	___	___
7. Remind the patient not to place toilet paper in the bedpan, specipan, or specimen container. Provide a waste bag for dirty paper.	___	___
8. Put on your gloves.	___	___
9. Help the patient clean the perineal area, if necessary.	___	___
10. Take the bedpan, urinal, or specipan to the bathroom.	___	___
11. If the patient's intake/output is being measured, measure and record the amount of urine.	___	___
12. Pour the urine into the specimen container. The container should be 3/4 full.	___	___
13. Place the lid on the specimen container.	___	___
14. Pour the remaining urine into the toilet.	___	___
15. Clean the equipment and store for the next use.	___	___
16. Discard the waste bag.	___	___
17. Remove your gloves.	___	___
18. Wash your hands.	___	___
19. Help the patient wash his or her hands.	___	___
20. Make the patient comfortable and place the signal cord within reach.	___	___

	Yes	No
21. Unscreen the patient.	___	___
22. Take the urine specimen to the nurse's station or the lab. Be sure to take the lab requisition slip with the specimen.	___	___
23. Wash your hands.	___	___
24. Report your observations to the nurse.	___	___

Procedure Completed ______________________ **Date** ______________

Notes ____

____

____

PROCEDURE

SP

COLLECTING A CLEAN-CATCH OR MIDSTREAM SAMPLE

Standard Precautions ☐ Handwashing ☐ Gloving ☐ Gowning ☐ Masking

Introductory Tasks ☐ Gather Equipment ☐ Identify/Introduce/Explain ☐ Provide Privacy

	Yes	No
6. Help the patient to the bathroom if the patient is able. Otherwise, perform the procedure while the patient is in bed.	___	___
7. Open the clean-catch urine kit. Remove the towelettes and the specimen container.	___	___
8. Put on your gloves.	___	___
9. Perform perineal care using the towelettes. Patients who are able can do this on their own. Remind the patient that each towelette should be used for only one wipe (from front to back). Women should keep their labia separated until the specimen is collected. An uncircumcised male should keep the foreskin retracted until the specimen is collected.	___	___
10. Ask the patient to urinate in the bedpan, urinal, specipan, or toilet.	___	___
11. Ask the patient to stop the stream.	___	___
12. Hold the specimen container under the patient. Note that patients who are able can do this on their own.	___	___
13. Ask the patient to start urinating again.	___	___
14. Ask the patient to stop urinating at the point at which the container is about 3/4 full.	___	___

	Yes	No
15. Remove the container and ask the patient to finish urinating.	___	___
16. Place the lid on the specimen container with your clean hand.	___	___
17. Help the patient clean the perineal area.	___	___
18. Take the bedpan, urinal, or specipan to the bathroom.	___	___
19. If the patient's intake/output is being measured, measure and record the amount of urine. Make sure you include the urine in the specimen container in your calculations.	___	___
20. Pour the remaining urine into the toilet.	___	___
21. Clean the equipment and store for the next use.	___	___
22. Remove your gloves.	___	___
23. Wash your hands.	___	___
24. Help the patient wash his or her hands.	___	___
25. Make the patient comfortable and place the signal cord within reach.	___	___
26. Unscreen the patient.	___	___
27. Take the urine specimen to the nurse's station or the lab. Be sure to take the lab requisition slip with the specimen.	___	___
28. Wash your hands.	___	___
29. Report your observations to the nurse.	___	___

Procedure Completed ______________________________ **Date** ______________________

Notes ____

____

____

PROCEDURE

COLLECTING A FRACTIONAL SAMPLE

Standard Precautions ☐ Handwashing ☐ Gloving ☐ Gowning ☐ Masking

Introductory Tasks ☐ Gather Equipment ☐ Identify/Introduce/Explain ☐ Provide Privacy

	Yes	No
5. Ask the patient to urinate in the bedpan, urinal, or specipan. If the patient is able, he or she can go to the bathroom to urinate and provide a sample in the specimen container.	___	___
6. Remind the patient not to place toilet paper in the bedpan or specipan. Provide a waste bag for dirty paper.	___	___
7. Put on your gloves.	___	___
8. Take the bedpan, urinal, or specipan to the bathroom.	___	___
9. If the patient's intake/output is being measured, measure and record the amount of urine.	___	___
10. Pour the urine into the specimen container. The container should be 3/4 full.	___	___
11. Test the urine in case a second sample cannot be obtained. Note on the specimen label that the test was done on the first sample.	___	___
12. Pour the remaining urine into the toilet.	___	___
13. Clean the equipment and store for the next use.	___	___
14. Discard the waste bag.	___	___
15. Remove your gloves.	___	___
16. Wash your hands.	___	___
17. Help the patient wash his or her hands.	___	___
18. Make the patient comfortable and place the signal cord within reach.	___	___
19. Unscreen the patient.	___	___
20. Return to the room in 20 to 30 minutes.	___	___
21. Repeat Steps 5 through 19.	___	___
22. Wash your hands.	___	___
23. Report the results of the tests and your observations to the nurse.	___	___

Procedure Completed ______________________ **Date** ______________

Notes ____

____

____

PROCEDURE

COLLECTING A 24-HOUR URINE SPECIMEN

Standard Precautions ☐ Handwashing ☐ Gloving ☐ Gowning ☐ Masking

Introductory Tasks ☐ Gather Equipment ☐ Identify/Introduce/Explain ☐ Provide Privacy

	Yes	No
6. Place the equipment in the patient's bathroom.	___	___
7. Write the patient's information on the urine collection container.	___	___
8. Place one of the 24-hour urine collection labels in the patient's bathroom. Place the other label near the bed.	___	___
9. Offer the patient the bedpan, urinal, or commode, or help the patient to the bathroom. Wear gloves if you need to help the patient.	___	___
10. Ask the patient to urinate. Discard this specimen. The 24-hour period begins after the patient urinates.	___	___
11. Write the time the test began and the time it will end on the labels and the specimen container.	___	___
12. Explain to the patient that he or she will use the bedpan, urinal, or specipan each time he or she urinates for the next 24 hours. Remind the patient not to have a bowel movement at the same time as he or she urinates.	___	___
13. After the patient urinates, pour the urine into the urine collection container using the funnel. Be careful not to spill any urine. Replace the container on ice or in the refrigerator.	___	___
14. At the end of the 24-hour period, ask the patient to urinate. Add the urine to the collection container. Remove your gloves.	___	___
15. Make the patient comfortable and place the signal cord within reach.	___	___
16. Clean and disinfect all the equipment. Store for the next use.	___	___
17. Remove the labels from the bed and bathroom.	___	___
18. Thank the patient for his or her cooperation.	___	___
19. Wash your hands.	___	___
20. Take the urine collection container to the nurse's station or the lab. Be sure to take the lab requisition slip with the specimen.	___	___
21. Wash your hands.	___	___
22. Report your observations to the nurse.	___	___

Procedure Completed ____________________ Date ____________________

Notes ____

____

____

PROCEDURE

COLLECTING URINE FROM AN INFANT OR TODDLER

Standard Precautions ☐ Handwashing ☐ Gloving ☐ Gowning ☐ Masking

Introductory Tasks ☐ Gather Equipment ☐ Identify/Introduce/Explain ☐ Provide Privacy

	Yes	No
7. Remove the child's diaper.	___	___
8. Clean the perineal area with water and sterile cotton balls. Dry the area.	___	___
9. Place the child on his or her back, with the knees flexed.	___	___
10. Remove the backing from the urine collector. Place the bag over the boy's penis or the girl's vulva. Do not cover the anus. Press the adhesive gently on the child's skin so the collector stays in place.	___	___
11. Diaper the child as usual.	___	___
12. Remove your gloves.	___	___
13. Make the child comfortable and provide for safety.	___	___
14. Unscreen the child.	___	___
15. Wash your hands.	___	___
16. Return periodically to check if the child has urinated. Open the diaper to check.	___	___
17. Once the child has urinated, provide privacy. Put on your gloves.	___	___
18. Remove the diaper.	___	___
19. Remove the urine collector.	___	___
20. Pour the contents into the specimen container. Cover it with the lid using your clean hand.	___	___
21. Discard the urine collector.	___	___
22. Provide perineal care to the child.	___	___
23. Put a clean diaper on the child.	___	___
24. Make the child comfortable and place the signal cord within reach.	___	___
25. Remove your gloves.	___	___

	Yes	No
26. Wash your hands.	___	___
27. Unscreen the child.	___	___
28. Place the label on the specimen container.	___	___
29. Discard disposable items.	___	___
30. Take the urine specimen to the nurse's station or the lab. Be sure to take the lab requisition slip with the specimen.	___	___
31. Wash your hands.	___	___
32. Report your observations to the nurse.	___	___

Procedure Completed ______________________ **Date** ______________________

Notes ____

____

____

PROCEDURE

TESTING URINE SAMPLES

Standard Precautions ☐ Handwashing ☐ Gloving ☐ Gowning ☐ Masking

Introductory Tasks ☐ Gather Equipment ☐ Identify/Introduce/Explain ☐ Provide Privacy

	Yes	No
6. Follow Procedure, Collecting a Fractional Sample, to collect a fractional urine specimen.	___	___
7. For Testape test:		
—Open the dispenser. Tear off about 1-1/2 inches of Testape.	___	___
—Dip 1/4 inch of Testape into the urine specimen. Remove the tape immediately.	___	___
—Hold the tape downward.	___	___
—Wait 60 seconds.	___	___
—Compare the darkest color on the tape to the color chart on the dispenser.	___	___
—Read the number that corresponds to the color. Record the number.	___	___
—Discard the used tape and the urine specimen.	___	___
8. For Clinitest:		
—Put paper towels over your work area.	___	___

	Yes	No
—Place a clean test tube in the holder.	___	___
—Rinse the medicine dropper with water and then draw urine into the dropper.	___	___
—Place 5 drops of urine in the clean test tube.	___	___
—Rinse the medicine dropper. Draw clean water in the medicine dropper and add 10 drops of water into the test tube.	___	___
—Drop one Clinitest tablet into the bottle cap and then into the test tube by tapping the Clinitest container gently so one tablet falls out. Do not let the tablet touch your skin.	___	___
—Do not touch the test tube.	___	___
—The contents of the test tube produces a boiling reaction.	___	___
—Wait 15 seconds after the boiling has stopped. Gently shake the test tube.	___	___
—Match the color of the liquid with the color chart on the Clinitest container. Record the corresponding number.	___	___
—Discard the test tube contents.	___	___
—Clean the test tube and medicine dropper and return them to the kit.	___	___
—Discard disposable equipment.	___	___
9. For Acetest:		
— Line the over-bed table with paper towels.	___	___
—Place one Acetest tablet on the paper towel by tapping one tablet into the bottle cap. Drop the tablet onto the paper towel without touching the tablet.	___	___
—Using a clean medicine dropper, place one drop of urine on the tablet.	___	___
—Wait 30 seconds.	___	___
—Compare the color of the tablet with the color chart on the side of the Acetest bottle.	___	___
—Read the result that corresponds to the color chart.	___	___
—Record the result.	___	___
—Discard the paper towels, Acetest tablet, and urine.	___	___
10. For Keto-Diastix test:		
—Remove a strip from the Keto-Diastix container. Cover the container immediately.	___	___
—Dip the two test areas into the urine specimen for 2 seconds.	___	___
—Remove the strip from the specimen. Tap the strip against the container to remove excess urine.	___	___
—Wait 15 seconds.	___	___
—Compare the area that was light pink to the color chart. This tests for ketones in the urine. Record the results.	___	___
—After 30 seconds, compare the area that was blue to the color chart. This tests for glucose in the urine. Record the results.	___	___

	Yes	No
—Discard the strip and specimen in a waste container.	___	___
11. Clean equipment and store for next use.	___	___
12. Remove your gloves.	___	___
13. Wash your hands.	___	___
14. Report the results and your observations to the nurse.	___	___

Procedure Completed ______________________ **Date** ______________________

Notes ____

____

____

PROCEDURE

STRAINING URINE FOR STONES

Standard Precautions ☐ Handwashing ☐ Gloving ☐ Gowning ☐ Masking

Introductory Tasks ☐ Gather Equipment ☐ Identify/Introduce/Explain ☐ Provide Privacy

	Yes	No
7. Offer the bedpan, urinal, or bedside commode, or assist the patient to the toilet to use the specipan.	___	___
8. After the patient has voided, remove and cover the bedpan, urinal, or bedside commode. Assist the patient with perineal care. If the patient was able to use the toilet, assist with perineal care and help the patient back to the room.	___	___
9. Help the patient wash his or her hands.	___	___
10. Make the patient comfortable and place the signal cord within reach.	___	___
11. Take the urine into the patient's bathroom.	___	___
12. Place the strainer or gauze over a specimen container.	___	___
13. Pour the urine into the strainer or gauze. Any stones, crystals, or particles will remain in the strainer or on the gauze.	___	___
14. Discard the urine.	___	___
15. Place the gauze or contents of the strainer in the specimen container. Cover the container.	___	___
16. Remove your gloves.	___	___

	Yes	No
17. Wash your hands.	___	___
18. Label the container.	___	___
19. Clean and store equipment for the next use.	___	___
20. Unscreen the patient.	___	___
21. Take the urine specimen to the nurse's station or the lab. Be sure to take the lab requisition slip with the specimen.	___	___
22. Wash your hands.	___	___
23. Report your observations to the nurse.	___	___

Procedure Completed ______________________ **Date** ______________

Notes ____

____

____

PROCEDURE

OBRA SP

COLLECTING A STOOL SAMPLE

Standard Precautions ☐ Handwashing ☐ Gloving ☐ Gowning ☐ Masking

Introductory Tasks ☐ Gather Equipment ☐ Identify/Introduce/Explain ☐ Provide Privacy

	Yes	No
7. Offer the bedpan or urinal for the patient to urinate in before producing a stool sample. Remove the bedpan and clean it.	___	___
8. Help the patient with toileting. Offer a different bedpan, specipan, or commode.	___	___
9. Remind the patient to put used toilet paper in the disposable bag.	___	___
10. Place the toilet paper and signal cord within reach.	___	___
11. Tell the patient to signal you when he or she is finished.	___	___
12. Remove your gloves. Wash your hands.	___	___
13. Leave the room.	___	___
14. Return to the room as soon as the patient signals. Knock before entering.	___	___
15. Put on your gloves.	___	___
16. Remove the bedpan from the patient and cover it.	___	___

	Yes	No
17. Assist the patient with perineal care.	___	___
18. Take the bedpan into the patient's bathroom.	___	___
19. Using the wooden blade, collect about 2 tablespoons of feces and place it in the specimen container.	___	___
20. Put the lid on the container, without touching the inside.	___	___
21. Cover the wooden blade with toilet paper and discard.	___	___
22. Empty and clean the bedpan or specipan.	___	___
23. Store equipment for the next use.	___	___
24. Remove your gloves.	___	___
25. Help the patient wash his or her hands.	___	___
26. Make the patient comfortable and place the signal cord within reach.	___	___
27. Place the label on the specimen container.	___	___
28. Place the specimen in a proper bag.	___	___
29. Wash your hands.	___	___
30. Unscreen the patient.	___	___
31. Take the stool specimen to the nurse's station or the lab. Be sure to take the lab requisition slip with the specimen.	___	___
32. Wash your hands.	___	___
33. Report your observations to the nurse.	___	___

Procedure Completed ______________________ **Date** ______________________

Notes ____

____

____

PROCEDURE

COLLECTING A HEMOCCULT SLIDE

Standard Precautions ☐ Handwashing ☐ Gloving ☐ Gowning ☐ Masking

Introductory Tasks ☐ Gather Equipment ☐ Identify/Introduce/Explain ☐ Provide Privacy

	Yes	No
8. Open the back of the test packet. There are two paper squares labeled A and B. The packet is designed so that you never directly touch the stool specimen.	___	___
9. Use the wooden blade to pick up a small amount of stool. Smear a small amount on the square labeled A.	___	___
10. Turn the wooden blade around and pick up another small amount of stool from a different part of the specimen. Smear a small amount on the square labeled B.	___	___
11. Close the packet.	___	___
12. Turn the packet over and open it. There will be two paper areas with stool under the paper. One test area is marked positive (+), and the other is marked negative (-).	___	___
13. Open the developer and place one drop on the positive area and one drop on the negative area.	___	___
14. Wait 10 seconds.	___	___
15. The positive test area should turn blue. This indicates that the test is working.	___	___
16. Place 2 more drops of developer on the positive and negative areas. Replace the cap on the developer.	___	___
17. Read the results in 1 minute.	___	___
18. If there is no color change, there is no occult blood in the stool. If the color on the negative area turns blue, there is occult blood in the stool.	___	___
19. Save the test packet to show the nurse the results.	___	___
20. Flush the remaining stool specimen down the toilet.	___	___
21. Discard the wooden blade.	___	___
22. Clean and disinfect the equipment.	___	___
23. Remove your gloves.	___	___
24. Wash your hands.	___	___
25. Store equipment for the next use. Return the developer to the nurse's station.	___	___
26. Make the patient comfortable and place the signal cord within reach.	___	___
27. Note the test results on the patient's chart.	___	___
28. Report the results and any observations to the nurse.	___	___

Procedure Completed ______________________ Date ______________

Notes ____

____

____

PROCEDURE

INSERTING A RECTAL TUBE

Standard Precautions ☐ Handwashing ☐ Gloving ☐ Gowning ☐ Masking

Introductory Tasks ☐ Gather Equipment ☐ Identify/Introduce/Explain ☐ Provide Privacy

	Yes	No
5. Raise the bed to a comfortable working level.	___	___
6. Lower the side rail, if appropriate.	___	___
7. Position the patient in the left Sims' position. Place the waterproof bed protector under the patient's buttocks.	___	___
8. Put on your gloves.	___	___
9. Lubricate 2 to 4 inches of the tip of the rectal tube.	___	___
10. Expose the anal area by lifting the edge of the bed linens.	___	___
11. Lift the upper buttock to expose the anus.	___	___
12. Ask the patient to take a deep breath.	___	___
13. As the patient exhales, gently insert the rectal tube 2 to 4 inches into the rectum. Stop if the patient complains of pain.	___	___
14. Tape the tubing to the lower buttock to hold it in place.	___	___
15. Position the flatus bag so it is on the bed behind the patient on the waterproof bed protector.	___	___
16. Remove your gloves.	___	___
17. Cover the patient.	___	___
18. Wash your hands.	___	___
19. Let the tube remain in place for 20 minutes.	___	___
20. Make the patient comfortable and place the signal cord within reach.	___	___
21. Leave the room.	___	___
22. Return in 20 minutes.	___	___
23. Put on your gloves.	___	___
	___	___

	Yes	No
24. Remove the tube and flatus bag and discard them.	___	___
25. Help the patient wipe the anal area.	___	___
26. Have the nurse check the abdominal distention.	___	___
27. Remove your gloves.	___	___
28. Wash your hands.	___	___
29. Make the patient comfortable and place the signal cord within reach.	___	___
30. Unscreen the patient.	___	___
31. Wash your hands.	___	___
32. Report your observations to the nurse.	___	___

Procedure Completed ______________________ **Date** ______________________

Notes ____

____

____

PROCEDURE

INSERTING A RECTAL SUPPOSITORY

Standard Precautions ☐ Handwashing ☐ Gloving ☐ Gowning ☐ Masking

Introductory Tasks ☐ Gather Equipment ☐ Identify/Introduce/Explain ☐ Provide Privacy

	Yes	No
5. Raise the bed to a comfortable working level.	___	___
6. Lower the side rail, if appropriate.	___	___
7. Place the bed protector under the patient's buttocks.	___	___
8. Position the patient in the left Sims' position.	___	___
9. Put on your gloves.	___	___
10. Open the suppository. Lubricate it with the lubricating jelly.	___	___
11. Use one hand to lift the top buttock.	___	___
12. Insert the suppository with the other hand. Gently push it in. Place the suppository past the rectal sphincter muscle.	___	___
13. Tell the patient to hold in the suppository for at least 20 minutes. You may need to briefly hold toilet paper against the anus.	___	___

	Yes	No
14. Wipe the patient's anus with the toilet paper. Discard the used paper.	___	___
15. Remove the bed protector.	___	___
16. In about 30 minutes the patient usually feels the urge to defecate. Offer the bedpan or bedside commode or take the patient to the toilet.	___	___
17. Remove your gloves. Make the patient comfortable and place the signal cord within reach.	___	___
18. Wash your hands.	___	___
19. Report your observations to the nurse.	___	___

Procedure Completed ______________________ **Date** ______________________

Notes ____

____

____

PROCEDURE

GIVING A CLEANSING ENEMA

Standard Precautions ☐ Handwashing ☐ Gloving ☐ Gowning ☐ Masking

Introductory Tasks ☐ Gather Equipment ☐ Identify/Introduce/Explain ☐ Provide Privacy

	Yes	No
5. Raise the bed to a comfortable working level.	___	___
6. Lower the side rail, if applicable.	___	___
7. Place the bed protector under the patient's buttocks.	___	___
8. Cover the patient with the bath blanket and fanfold the top linens to the foot of the bed.	___	___
9. Place the IV pole next to the bed. Adjust the pole so the enema bag will be 12 inches above the anus or 18 inches above the mattress.	___	___
10. Place the bedpan or commode within reach.	___	___
11. Raise the side rail (if appropriate) and go to the patient's bathroom.	___	___
12. Open the disposable enema kit. Attach the tubing to the enema bag. Close the clamp on the tubing.	___	___
13. Fill the measuring container with the prescribed amount of solution. Add the ingredients as ordered by the patient's doctor.	___	___

	Yes	No
14. Measure the temperature of the solution using the bath thermometer. The solution should be 105° F.	___	___
15. Pour the solution into the enema bag. Shake the solution gently to mix it.	___	___
16. Open the clamp and run a small amount of the solution into the sink. Reclamp. This removes the air from the tubing.	___	___
17. Return to the patient.	___	___
18. Hang the enema bag on the IV pole.	___	___
19. Lower the side rail, if appropriate.	___	___
20. Position the patient in the left Sims' position.	___	___
21. Put on your gloves.	___	___
22. Expose the patient's anal area by lifting the top buttock.	___	___
23. Lubricate 2 to 4 inches of the tip of the enema tubing with the lubricant.	___	___
24. Ask the patient to take a deep breath.	___	___
25. Gently insert the tip of the tubing 2 to 4 inches into the rectum as the patient exhales. Stop if you feel resistance or the patient complains of pain.	___	___
26. Unclamp the tubing and slowly administer the enema. Hold the enema tube in place as you administer the solution. Clamp the tubing to stop the enema if the patient experiences cramping. Resume when the cramping stops.	___	___
27. Clamp the tubing if the patient has the urge to defecate.	___	___
28. When most of the solution has flowed into the rectum, close the clamp.	___	___
29. Slowly withdraw the tubing from the rectum. Wrap the tip of the tubing with toilet paper. Discard it.	___	___
30. Encourage the patient to hold the solution as long as possible or help hold the buttocks together, if necessary.	___	___
31. When the patient is ready to defecate, help him or her to the toilet or assist with the bedpan or commode. Remind the patient not to flush the toilet.	___	___
32. Place the signal cord and toilet paper within reach.	___	___
33. Remove your gloves.	___	___
34. Wash your hands.	___	___
35. Leave the room if the patient can be alone.	___	___
36. Return immediately when the patient signals. Knock before entering the room.	___	___
37. Wash your hands and put on your gloves.	___	___
38. Observe the feces for amount, odor, color, and character.	___	___
39. Remove the bedpan or assist the patient back to bed.	___	___
40. Provide perineal care as necessary.	___	___
41. Cover the patient with the top linens and remove the bath blanket. Remove the bed protector.	___	___
42. Make the patient comfortable and place the signal cord within reach.	___	___

	Yes	No
43. Empty, clean, and disinfect the bedpan or commode. Flush the toilet after the nurse looks at the output.	___	___
44. Store equipment for the next use.	___	___
45. Remove your gloves.	___	___
46. Help the patient wash his or her hands.	___	___
47. Unscreen the patient.	___	___
48. Place soiled linen in the hamper.	___	___
49. Wash your hands.	___	___
50. Report your observations to the nurse, such as the type of enema used, how much solution was taken, characteristics of the stool, and how the patient tolerated the procedure.	___	___

Procedure Completed ______________________ **Date** ______________

Notes ____

____

____

PROCEDURE

GIVING SPECIAL TYPES OF ENEMAS

Standard Precautions ☐ Handwashing ☐ Gloving ☐ Gowning ☐ Masking

Introductory Tasks ☐ Gather Equipment ☐ Identify/Introduce/Explain ☐ Provide Privacy

	Yes	No
5. Raise the bed to a comfortable working level.	___	___
6. Lower the side rail, if appropriate.	___	___
7. Place the bed protector under the patient's buttocks.	___	___
8. Cover the patient with the bath blanket and fanfold the top linens to the foot of the bed.	___	___
9. Place the bedpan or commode within reach.	___	___
10. Position the patient in the left Sims' position.	___	___
11. Put on your gloves.	___	___
12. Expose the patient's anal area by lifting the top buttock.	___	___
13. Remove the cap from the enema. Lubricate the tip with lubricating jelly.	___	___

	Yes	No
14. Ask the patient to take a deep breath while you perform the next step.	___	___
15. Gently insert the tip of the enema 2 inches into the rectum as the patient exhales. Stop if you feel resistance or the patient complains of pain.	___	___
16. Squeeze and roll the plastic bottle gently until all the solution enters the rectum.	___	___
17. Remove the tube from the rectum and dispose of it in the box.	___	___
18. When giving an oil retention enema, encourage the patient to hold the solution for the specified time, usually 30 to 60 minutes, before defecating. When giving a cleansing enema, encourage the patient to hold the solution until he or she feels the urge to defecate. Help hold the buttocks together, if necessary.	___	___
19. When the patient is ready to defecate, help him or her to the toilet or assist with the bedpan or commode. Remind the patient not to flush the toilet.	___	___
20. Place the signal cord and toilet paper within reach.	___	___
21. Remove your gloves.	___	___
22. Wash your hands.	___	___
23. Leave the room if the patient can be alone.	___	___
24. Return immediately when the patient signals. Knock before entering the room.	___	___
25. Wash your hands and put on your gloves.	___	___
26. Observe the feces for amount, odor, color, and character. Save it if the nurse has asked to look at it.	___	___
27. Remove the bedpan or assist the patient back to bed.	___	___
28. Provide perineal care as necessary.	___	___
29. Cover the patient with the top linens and remove the bath blanket. Remove the bed protector.	___	___
30. Make the patient comfortable and place the signal cord within reach.	___	___
31. Empty, clean, and disinfect the bedpan or commode. Flush the toilet.	___	___
32. Store equipment for the next use.	___	___
33. Remove your gloves.	___	___
34. Help the patient wash his or her hands.	___	___
35. Unscreen the patient.	___	___
36. Place soiled linen in the hamper.	___	___
37. Wash your hands.	___	___
38. Report your observations to the nurse.	___	___

Procedure Completed ______________________________ **Date** ____________________

Notes ____

____

____

PROCEDURE

CHANGING A COLOSTOMY APPLIANCE

Standard Precautions ☐ Handwashing ☐ Gloving ☐ Gowning ☐ Masking

Introductory Tasks ☐ Gather Equipment ☐ Identify/Introduce/Explain ☐ Provide Privacy

	Yes	No
5. Raise the bed to a comfortable working level.	___	___
6. Lower the side rail, if appropriate.	___	___
7. Line the over-bed table with paper towels.	___	___
8. Place the bed protector under the patient's buttocks.	___	___
9. Cover the patient with the bath blanket and fanfold the top linens to the foot of the bed.	___	___
10. Remove the belt. Discard it in a waste bag.	___	___
11. Gently disconnect the appliance from the patient. Place the appliance in a bedpan.	___	___
12. Wipe around the stoma with toilet paper. Remove any feces or drainage. Discard the toilet paper in a bedpan or waste bag.	___	___
13. Cover the bedpan and take it into the patient's bathroom.	___	___
14. Note the color, odor, amount, and character of the feces. Empty the bedpan into the toilet. Discard the appliance in the waste bag.	___	___
15. Fill the wash basin with warm water. Place it on the over-bed table.	___	___
16. Clean the skin around the stoma with warm water. Use soap or a cleaning agent, according to facility policy. Rinse well and dry.	___	___
17. Apply the karaya powder, ring, or other skin barrier.	___	___
18. Place the deodorant in the appliance.	___	___
19. Remove the backing on the new appliance. Center it over the stoma and seal it to the skin. You can press gently to make sure it is sealed.	___	___
20. Remove the bed protector.	___	___
21. Discard the waste bag.	___	___
22. Remove your gloves.	___	___
23. Make the patient comfortable and place the signal cord within reach.	___	___
24. Unscreen the patient.	___	___
25. Clean and disinfect the equipment.	___	___
26. Store it for the next use.	___	___
27. Wash your hands.	___	___
28. Report your observations to the nurse.	___	___

Procedure Completed ______________________ **Date** ______________________

Notes ____

____

____

PROCEDURE

HELPING THE ILEOSTOMY PATIENT

Standard Precautions ☐ Handwashing ☐ Gloving ☐ Gowning ☐ Masking

Introductory Tasks ☐ Gather Equipment ☐ Identify/Introduce/Explain ☐ Provide Privacy

	Yes	No
6. Help the patient out of bed, into the bathroom, and onto the toilet.	___	___
7. Put on your gloves.	___	___
8. Direct the appliance into the toilet. Remove the clamp. This empties the contents of the appliance into the toilet.	___	___
9. Wipe the end of the appliance with toilet paper. Some patients can do this themselves.	___	___
10. Note the color, odor, amount, and character of the feces.	___	___
11. Place a few drops of the solvent in the medicine dropper and apply it to the skin around the appliance. The appliance will loosen.	___	___
12. Gently remove the appliance.	___	___
13. Cover the stoma with the gauze.	___	___
14. Wet a cotton ball with the solvent and wipe around the stoma.	___	___
15. Clean the skin around the stoma with water. Some facilities also use soap or a cleansing agent. Rinse well and dry.	___	___
16. Remove the gauze.	___	___
17. Place the karaya ring around the stoma.	___	___
18. Put the deodorant in the appliance.	___	___
19. Clamp the bottom of the appliance and attach the appliance to the karaya ring.	___	___
20. Remove your gloves and wash your hands.	___	___
21. Help the patient to wash his or her hands.	___	___
22. Make the patient comfortable and place the signal cord within reach.	___	___
23. Unscreen the patient.	___	___

	Yes	No
24. Put on clean gloves.	___	___
25. Clean the appliance with the soft brush.	___	___
26. Allow the appliance to dry.	___	___
27. Remove your gloves.	___	___
28. Store equipment for the next use.	___	___
29. Wash your hands.	___	___
30. Report your observations to the nurse.	___	___

Procedure Completed ______________________ **Date** ______________________

Notes ____

____

____

PROCEDURE

COLLECTING AND PRESERVING A SPUTUM SAMPLE

Standard Precautions ☐ Handwashing ☐ Gloving ☐ Gowning ☐ Masking

Introductory Tasks ☐ Gather Equipment ☐ Identify/Introduce/Explain ☐ Provide Privacy

	Yes	No
7. If the patient has eaten recently, ask the patient to rinse out his or her mouth.	___	___
8. Give the patient the specimen container.	___	___
9. Instruct the patient to take several deep breaths and then cough deeply from the lungs to bring up sputum. The patient should cover his or her mouth and nose with a tissue while coughing.	___	___
10. The patient may need to cough several times to bring up enough sputum. One to two tablespoons of sputum is needed for the specimen.	___	___
11. Instruct the patient to spit directly into the specimen container.	___	___
12. Put the lid on the container immediately after collection.	___	___
13. Place the completed label on the container.	___	___
14. Remove your gloves.	___	___
15. Wash your hands.	___	___
16. Make the patient comfortable and place the signal cord within reach.	___	___

	Yes	No
17. Unscreen the patient.	___	___
18. Take the sputum specimen to the nurse's station or the lab. Be sure to take the lab requisition slip with the specimen.	___	___
19. Wash your hands.	___	___
20. Report the following to the nurse: • Date and time of sputum collection • Appearance of sputum • Time the specimen was sent to the lab • Any unusual observations	___	___

Procedure Completed ______________________ **Date** ______________________

Notes ____

____

____

CHAPTER 23

CARING FOR PATIENTS WITH CHRONIC ILLNESSES

STUDY OBJECTIVES

Chronic illnesses occur gradually and then last a long time, usually more than three months. Some patients with chronic illnesses require constant care. Others require some help with the activities of daily living, but are generally able to take care of their own needs.

- Patients with diabetes require special attention to the skin and feet to avoid problems associated with poor circulation. The patients must follow a strict special diet and must be observed for symptoms of hyperglycemia or hypoglycemia.
- Patients with kidney failure require monitoring for fluid and food intake. Areas that are involved in dialysis should be kept clean.
- Patients with cancer need to be kept as free of infection as possible. They also need encouragement to eat, rest, and express their feelings.
- Patients with AIDS need to be kept as free of infection as possible. They need to be encouraged to eat, to perform range-of-motion exercises, and to be given emotional support.
- Patients who have had a stroke should be kept clean. They should be encouraged to participate fully in their own rehabilitation and to be as independent as possible.
- Observe patients with CHF for any changes that may indicate trouble. Also, positioning of patients with CHF is important for comfort.
- Because Parkinson's disease involves loss of control over movements, encourage patients to use special devices to maintain as much independence as possible.

KNOW YOUR TERMS

In the space provided, write the letter of the definition that best fits the numbered term.

__ 1. angina pectoris
__ 2. aphasia
__ 3. cancer
__ 4. carcinogen
__ 5. carcinoma
__ 6. cardiovascular
__ 7. chemotherapy
__ 8. congestive heart failure (CHF)
__ 9. diabetic coma
__10. gangrene
__11. glucose
__12. HIV wasting syndrome
__13. hyperglycemia
__14. hypoglycemia
__15. insulin
__16. insulin shock
__17. kidney dialysis
__18. kidney (renal) failure
__19. radiation
__20. syndrome

a. A cancer-causing substance.
b. The treatment of disease by chemical means (said especially of cancer treatment).
c. A form of sugar.
d. A coma due to severe glucose imbalance.
e. An abnormal decrease of glucose in the blood.
f. Any of various diseases characterized by malignant tumors that invade surrounding tissues.
g. A pancreatic hormone crucial to the regulation of carbohydrates in the body; a synthetic version of this hormone used in the treatment of diabetes.
h. A procedure for cleaning the blood of a patient with kidney failure, using a machine.
i. A method of treating diseases (as cancer) by exposing the diseased area to a form of energy.
j. The presence of too much insulin in the body, causing coma.
k. The loss of kidney function.
l. A malignant tumor.
m. A loss of 10 percent or more of the body's weight in a short time due to symptoms of AIDS.
n. A group of signs and symptoms that together form a particular condition or abnormality.
o. Of the heart and blood vessels.
p. An abnormally high level of glucose in the blood.
q. Death of a body part or area due to loss or severe lessening of blood supply to that area.
r. Heart failure due to inadequately circulating blood.
s. Severe pain in the chest due to heart disease.
t. Inability or impaired ability to speak.

TEST YOUR KNOWLEDGE

Write the word(s) that best completes the statement.

1. Diabetes mellitus results when the body cannot change ____________ into energy.

2. ______________ is a condition that occurs when blood glucose levels are below normal.
3. ______________ occurs when there is too much glucose in the blood.
4. People who have kidney failure usually need______________ ______________ to remove waste products from their blood.
5. A malignant tumor is called a ______________.
6. A substance that causes cancer is called a ______________.
7. The HIV virus usually leads to the development of ______________.
8. A ______________ ______________ is also known as a stroke.
9. ______________ ______________ ______________ is caused by a weak heart that cannot pump strongly enough.
10. Patients with ______________ ______________ gradually lose control over movement.

THINK ABOUT THE ISSUES

1. What are some of the health risks of stroke? How does your lifestyle help you avoid a stroke?
2. Some people with chronic illnesses lose their will to live. How can nursing assistants encourage them to enjoy as much of life as they can?

CHECK YOUR SKILLS

In the following procedure checklists, check each task box that applies and answer yes or no to each step you have completed. If possible, have your instructor sign off when you have completed a procedure.

PROCEDURE

SP

TESTING URINE FOR (A) GLUCOSE AND (B) ACETONE

Standard Precautions ☐ Handwashing ☐ Gloving ☐ Gowning ☐ Masking

Introductory Tasks ☐ Gather Equipment ☐ Identify/Introduce/Explain ☐ Provide Privacy

	Yes	No
2. Take a test strip and close the bottle.	___	___
3. Dip one end of the test strip into the urine.	___	___
4. Remove the strip immediately and hold it horizontally.	___	___
5. Follow the manufacturer's instructions as to how long to wait before reading the strip.	___	___

	Yes	No
6. Compare the strip to the color chart on the bottle. Do not touch the bottle's label with the wet strip.	___	___
7. Dispose of the strip in a biohazard container and flush the urine specimen, unless you have other instructions.	___	___
8. Remove gloves and properly dispose of them.	___	___
9. Report the following to your supervisor: • That the test is complete • Your findings • Any unusual observations	___	___

Procedure Completed ______________________ **Date** ______________________

Notes ____

____

____

CHAPTER 24

Caring for the Surgical Patient

Study Objectives

Patients need preoperative care to prepare them for surgery and postoperative care to help them recover from surgery.

- ▲ Nursing assistants help admit the patient to the preoperative unit by measuring and recording vital signs, collecting urine samples, and administering enemas or any other prescribed procedure. They also shave patients if ordered by the nurse or doctor.
- ▲ Postoperative procedures include monitoring vital signs and helping with breathing and leg exercises as the patient wakes up from the anesthesia.
- ▲ Ambulatory and outpatient surgery is surgery performed without an overnight hospital stay.

KNOW YOUR TERMS

In the space provided, write the letter of the definition that best fits the numbered term.

__ 1. ambulatory surgery	a. Collapse of part or all of a lung.
__ 2. anesthesia	b. A mass that blocks blood in a vessel.
__ 3. atelectasis	c. Surgery that takes place on the same day the patient is released.
__ 4. embolus	d. Another name for ambulatory surgery.
__ 5. outpatient surgery	e. Agent for producing loss of sensation, usually given prior to surgery.
__ 6. same-day surgery	f. The use of manual procedures to treat diseases, injuries, or deformities.
__ 7. surgery	g. A blood clot in a blood vessel.
__ 8. thrombus	h. Surgery not requiring a hospital stay.

TEST YOUR KNOWLEDGE

Write the word(s) that best completes the statement.

1. The _____________ period begins when the surgical patient is admitted to the hospital.
2. Patients sign _____________ forms to give permission for a surgical procedure to be performed.
3. _____________ anesthesia puts the patient to sleep.
4. _____________ anesthesia blocks sensation to a defined area.
5. _____________ care begins when the patient returns to the nursing unit.
6. Vital signs are taken every _____________ minutes for the first hour after surgery.
7. One complication of surgery may be _____________, an infection in the lung.
8. _____________ is collapse of part of the lung.
9. A blood clot is called a _____________.
10. A blood clot that has broken loose and is traveling through the bloodstream is called an _____________.

THINK ABOUT THE ISSUES

1. Every surgery involves risks. Why do you think it is important for patients to understand those risks?
2. Pain medication is often needed after surgery during recuperation. Many pain medications can now be controlled by the patient. Do you think this is a good idea? Why or why not?

▲ CHECK YOUR SKILLS

In the following procedure checklists, check each task box that applies and answer yes or no to each step you have completed. If possible, have your instructor sign off when you have completed a procedure.

PROCEDURE

SHAVING THE PREOPERATIVE PATIENT

Standard Precautions ☐ Handwashing ☐ Gloving ☐ Gowning ☐ Masking

Introductory Tasks ☐ Gather Equipment ☐ Identify/Introduce/Explain ☐ Provide Privacy

	Yes	No
6. Make sure your lighting is good.	___	___
7. Raise the bed to the highest level.	___	___
8. Place the bath blanket over the patient and then fanfold the top linens to the foot of the bed.	___	___
9. Position the patient so the area to be shaved is in reach.	___	___
10. Place the bed protector under the patient.	___	___
11. Open the prep kit. Place the supplies on the over-bed table.	___	___
12. Drape the patient with the disposable drape.	___	___
13. Put on your gloves.	___	___
14. Dip the sponge in the water. Apply soap to the skin with the sponge and work up a good lather.	___	___
15. Hold the skin taut.	___	___
16. Shave in the direction the hair grows. Use short strokes, rinsing the razor often.	___	___
17. Wash the area with soap and water. Pat dry.	___	___
18. Make sure the area is free from any hair growth, cuts, and nicks.	___	___
19. Remove the drape and waterproof pad.	___	___
20. Remove your gloves.	___	___
21. Cover the patient with the bed linens and remove the bath blanket.	___	___
22. Lower the bed.	___	___
23. Make the patient comfortable and place the signal cord within reach.	___	___
24. Discard the used equipment. Place soiled linen in the hamper.	___	___
25. Open the screen.	___	___

	Yes	No
26. Wash your hands.	___	___
27. Record on the preoperative checklist that the skin prep was completed.	___	___
28. Report the following to the nurse: • Procedure was completed and the area prepped • Any cuts or nicks on the skin • Any unusual observations	___	___

Procedure Completed ______________________ **Date** ______________________

Notes ______________________

____

____

PROCEDURE

SP

ASSISTING THE PATIENT WITH DEEP-BREATHING AND COUGHING EXERCISES

Standard Precautions ☐ Handwashing ☐ Gloving ☐ Gowning ☐ Masking

Introductory Tasks ☐ Gather Equipment ☐ Identify/Introduce/Explain ☐ Provide Privacy

	Yes	No
5. Help the patient into a semi-Fowler's position.	___	___
6. A patient who has had abdominal surgery can hold a pillow over the abdomen to splint the incision.	___	___
7. Put on your gloves.	___	___
8. Ask the patient to place his or her hands on the sides of the rib cage or over the incision site.	___	___
9. Ask the patient to take a deep breath, hold it for 3 to 5 seconds, and slowly exhale. The patient should exhale through pursed lips.	___	___
10. Repeat the exercise until the patient reaches the number the nurse specified. If the patient is too exhausted to complete the specified number, report this to the nurse.	___	___
11. Help the patient cough. Ask the patient to interlace his or her fingers over the incision, or to hold a pillow against the incision.	___	___
12. Ask the patient to take a deep breath and cough forcefully two times.	___	___
13. Pass the patient tissues if any secretions come up with the coughs.	___	___

	Yes	No
14. Help the patient into a new, comfortable position.	___	___
15. Make the patient comfortable and place the signal cord within reach.	___	___
16. Discard used tissues. Store the pillow for next use.	___	___
17. Open the screen.	___	___
18. Remove your gloves.	___	___
19. Wash your hands.	___	___
20. Report the following to the nurse: • The number of times the patient performed each exercise • How the patient tolerated the procedure • Type and amount of any sputum coughed up	___	___

Procedure Completed ______________________ **Date** ______________

Notes ____

____

____

PROCEDURE

TURNING THE POSTOPERATIVE PATIENT

Standard Precautions ☐ Handwashing ☐ Gloving ☐ Gowning ☐ Masking

Introductory Tasks ☐ Gather Equipment ☐ Identify/Introduce/Explain ☐ Provide Privacy

	Yes	No
5. Raise the bed to the highest level.	___	___
6. Go to one side of the patient's bed. Your helper should stand on the other side.	___	___
7. Remove the existing supporting pillows.	___	___
8. The patient can hold a pillow over the incision for support if he or she is able.	___	___
9. Lower the side rails (if applicable).	___	___
10. Both you and your helper should place one hand near the patient's shoulder and the other hand on the buttocks.	___	___
11. Gently roll the patient onto his or her back.	___	___
12. Place your hands on the shoulders and buttocks or hips.	___	___
13. Gently roll the patient on his or her side.	___	___
14. Provide support with extra pillows.	___	___

	Yes	No
15. Lower the bed.	___	___
16. Make the patient comfortable and place the signal cord within reach.	___	___
17. Wash your hands.	___	___
18. Open the screen.	___	___
19. Report your observations to the nurse.	___	___

Procedure Completed ______________________ **Date** ______________________

Notes ____

____

____

PROCEDURE

HELPING THE PATIENT PERFORM LEG EXERCISES

Standard Precautions ☐ Handwashing ☐ Gloving ☐ Gowning ☐ Masking

Introductory Tasks ☐ Gather Equipment ☐ Identify/Introduce/Explain ☐ Provide Privacy

	Yes	No
5. Raise the bed to a comfortable working height.	___	___
6. Cover the patient's abdomen with a bath blanket and fanfold the top linens to the foot of the bed.	___	___
7. Help the patient to lie on his or her back, with the head supported with a pillow.	___	___
8. Instruct the patient to hold a pillow over the incision site to splint it.	___	___
9. Instruct the patient to do the following exercises. A weak patient may need your help. The patient should perform 3 to 5 repetitions of each exercise. • Rotate each ankle in circular movements. • Flex the toes up towards the knee; then point each foot. • Bend and extend each knee. • Bend and extend each hip.	___	___
10. Cover the patient and remove the bath blanket.	___	___
11. Lower the bed.	___	___
12. Make the patient comfortable and place the signal cord within reach.	___	___

	Yes	No
13. Wash your hands.	___	___
14. Report the following to the nurse: • Number of repetitions of each exercise accomplished • How the patient tolerated the procedure	___	___

Procedure Completed ______________________ **Date** ______________________

Notes ____

____

____

CHAPTER 25

EXAMINATIONS AND THERAPIES

STUDY OBJECTIVES

In some work situations, nursing assistants prepare patients for examinations. This may include gathering equipment, taking routine samples, draping and positioning the patient, and helping during and after the examination is complete. Nursing assistants provide various hot and cold therapies as directed by the nurse.

- ▲ Nursing assistants position and drape patients, take needed samples, and gather equipment.
- ▲ During an examination, nursing assistants may hand equipment to the examiner, label specimens, and clean and store equipment.
- ▲ Heat therapies include wet soaks, warm packs, sitz baths, heat lamps, aquamatic pads, and dry heat.
- ▲ Cold therapies include soaks, compresses, ice bags, sponge baths, and cold baths.
- ▲ Bandages, dressings, and binders are used to stop bleeding and to cover wounds.

KNOW YOUR TERMS

In the space provided, write the letter of the definition that best fits the numbered term.

__ 1. aquamatic pad	a. A piece of material used to apply pressure to a body part or wound.
__ 2. compress	b. Heat therapy that does not include moisture.
__ 3. cyanosis	c. Another name for compress.
__ 4. dry heat therapy	d. Any therapy that uses warm or hot water to provide heat.
__ 5. moist heat therapy	e. A type of heat therapy where the patient's pelvic region is immersed in warm water.
__ 6. pack	f. A type of heating pad through which warm water flows.
__ 7. sitz bath	g. The application of cool, moist cloths to the body to cool a patient with fever. Also, a bed bath, especially for an infant.
__ 8. sponge bath	h. A purplish or bluish discoloration of the skin or nails due to insufficient oxygen in the blood.

TEST YOUR KNOWLEDGE

Write the word(s) that best completes the statement.

1. A ______________ is a folded and moistened cloth placed over a small area of the body.
2. A warm ______________ is for larger areas of the body.
3. An ______________ ______________ is an electric heating pad composed of tubes filled with water.
4. Cold therapy ______________ blood flow.
5. Heat therapy ______________ blood flow.
6. ______________ ______________ are given to reduce high fever.
7. Elastic bandages may be used to ______________ an injured limb.
8. Bluish fingernails are a sign of ______________.
9. The patient's pelvic region is immersed in water during a ______________ ______________.
10. Dressings are usually made of ______________.

THINK ABOUT THE ISSUES

1. Waiting in an examination room can be a frightening experience. How can you help patients relax?
2. Heat therapy relaxes muscles and promotes healing. Cold therapy decreases swelling and lessens blood flow. Which do you think would most likely be used immediately after a fall? Why?

CHECK YOUR SKILLS

In the following procedure checklists, check each task box that applies and answer yes or no to each step you have completed. If possible, have your instructor sign off when you have completed a procedure.

PROCEDURE

PREPARING A PATIENT FOR AN EXAMINATION

Standard Precautions ☐ Handwashing ☐ Gloving ☐ Gowning ☐ Masking

Introductory Tasks ☐ Gather Equipment ☐ Identify/Introduce/Explain ☐ Provide Privacy

Step	Yes	No
5. Ask the patient to urinate. Help the patient into and out of the bathroom, if necessary. If the patient is bedridden, provide a bedpan. Collect urine, if indicated.	___	___
6. If the examination is not taking place in the patient's room, transport the patient to the examination room.	___	___
7. Ask the patient to remove all clothing and put on an examining gown with the opening in the front. If the patient needs assistance, stay and help. If the patient does not need assistance, leave the room while the patient undresses.	___	___
8. Help the patient get on the examination table. Have a stool available.	___	___
9. Raise the bed or examination table to the highest level.	___	___
10. Assist the patient in assuming the position desired by the examiner.	___	___
11. Arrange appropriate draping.	___	___
12. Place a bed protector under the buttocks.	___	___
13. Untie the examination gown.	___	___
14. Tell the examiner the patient is ready.	___	___

Procedure Completed ______________________ **Date** ______________

Notes ____

____

____

PROCEDURE

ASSISTING IN AN EXAMINATION

Standard Precautions ☐ Handwashing ☐ Gloving ☐ Gowning ☐ Masking

Introductory Tasks ☐ Gather Equipment ☐ Identify/Introduce/Explain ☐ Provide Privacy

Step	Yes	No
5. When the examiner lets you know the position he or she wants the patient to assume, explain that position to the patient.	___	___
6. Help the patient get into the position, if necessary.	___	___
7. Hand equipment and supplies to the examiner when requested.	___	___
8. Assist with repositioning the patient when necessary.	___	___
9. When the examination is complete, offer to help the patient get dressed. Ask if the patient is dizzy or lightheaded. If not, help the patient to a standing position.	___	___
10. Transport the patient back to his or her room.	___	___
11. Clean all equipment and return it to its storage location.	___	___
12. Wash your hands.	___	___

Procedure Completed ____________________ **Date** ____________________

Notes ____

____

____

PROCEDURE

APPLYING MOIST HEAT

Standard Precautions ☐ Handwashing ☐ Gloving ☐ Gowning ☐ Masking

Introductory Tasks ☐ Gather Equipment ☐ Identify/Introduce/Explain ☐ Provide Privacy

	Yes	No
5. Before applying the compress, place it under an ultraviolet light for 10 minutes.	___	___
6. Provide privacy.	___	___
7. Place the moisture-proof mattress protector under the area of the body you will bc treating.	___	___
8. Open the compress.	___	___
9. Using the foil wrap, apply the compress to the site. Do not delay; you must apply the compress while it is warm.	___	___
10. Cover the compress with the towel.	___	___
11. Place ties or rolled gauze over the towel to hold it in place.	___	___
12. Leave the compress in place for 20 to 30 minutes, but check the area every 5 minutes for signs of irritation or redness. Ask the patient if there is any pain or numbness. If there are any signs, remove the compress and tell the nurse right away.	___	___
13. During the treatment, check to be sure the compress is still warm. If it cools, apply another compress.	___	___
14. After 20 minutes, remove the ties or gauze, towel, and compress.	___	___
15. Use the towel to pat dry the site.	___	___
16. Check to make sure the patient is comfortable and that the body is aligned properly.	___	___
17. Make sure the signal light is within the patient's reach.	___	___
18. Open the screen.	___	___
19. Clean the equipment and return it to storage. Place soiled towels and linens in the laundry.	___	___
20. Wash your hands.	___	___
21. Record your observations and report anything unusual to the nurse: • Time of application • Site and length of application • How the patient tolerated the procedure • The condition of the skin	___	___

Procedure Completed ______________________________ **Date** ____________________

Notes ____

____

____

PROCEDURE

USING A HEAT LAMP

Standard Precautions ☐ Handwashing ☐ Gloving ☐ Gowning ☐ Masking

Introductory Tasks ☐ Gather Equipment ☐ Identify/Introduce/Explain ☐ Provide Privacy

	Yes	No
5. Turn on the lamp and give it ample time to warm up.	___	___
6. Provide privacy.	___	___
7. Uncover the part of the body that needs treatment.	___	___
8. Fanfold top linens down to the foot of the bed.	___	___
9. Place a bath blanket over the patient. Make sure the parts of the body not being treated are covered.	___	___
10. Use the tape measure or ruler to measure the distance from the bulb to the site.	___	___
11. Place the lamp an appropriate distance from the site: • 25 watt bulb—14 inches • 40 watt bulb—18 inches • 60 watt bulb—24 inches	___	___
12. The heat lamp is normally applied for 5 to 20 minutes. Check the area every 5 minutes for signs of blistering or redness. Ask the patient if there is any pain, burning, or numbness. If there are any signs, discontinue treatment and tell the nurse right away.	___	___
13. Remove the lamp after the prescribed number of minutes for the treatment have elapsed.	___	___
14. Return top linens to their proper position and remove the bath blanket.	___	___
15. Check to make sure the patient is comfortable and that the body is aligned properly.	___	___
16. Make sure the signal light is within the patient's reach.	___	___
17. Open the screen.	___	___
18. Clean the equipment and return it to storage.	___	___
19. Wash your hands.	___	___

	Yes	No
20. Record your observations and report any unusual signs to the nurse: • Time of application • Site and length of application • Distance between bulb and patient • How the patient tolerated the procedure • The condition of the skin	___	___

Procedure Completed ______________________ **Date** ______________

Notes ____

____

____

PROCEDURE

USING AN AQUAMATIC PAD

Standard Precautions ☐ Handwashing ☐ Gloving ☐ Gowning ☐ Masking

Introductory Tasks ☐ Gather Equipment ☐ Identify/Introduce/Explain ☐ Provide Privacy

	Yes	No
6. Uncover the part of the body that needs treatment.	___	___
7. Fanfold top linens down to the foot of the bed.	___	___
8. Place a bath blanket over the patient. Make sure the parts of the body not being treated are covered.	___	___
9. Check to be sure the pad has no leaks and that the cord and plug are in good condition. Fill the unit two-thirds full with distilled water.	___	___
10. Place the pad in its flannel cover.	___	___
11. Set the correct temperature with the key. Plug in the unit. Allow time for the water to reach the desired temperature, as instructed by the nurse.	___	___
12. Place the container on the bedside stand or over-bed table.	___	___
13. Make sure the pad and hoses are level with the heating unit.	___	___
14. Gently place the pad over the treatment area. (Be sure the patient does not lie on top of the pad.) Hold it in place with ties or gauze. Do not use pins.	___	___
15. During treatment, check the area regularly for signs of blistering, swelling, or redness. Ask the patient if there is any pain, burning, or numbness. If any signs or symptoms appear, discontinue treatment and tell the nurse right away.	___	___
16. After the specified treatment time, remove the pad.	___	___

	Yes	No
17. Check to make sure the patient is comfortable and that the body is aligned.	___	___
18. Make sure the signal light is within the patient's reach.	___	___
19. Open the screen.	___	___
20. Clean the equipment and return it to storage.	___	___
21. Wash your hands.	___	___
22. Record your observations and report anything unusual to the nurse: • Time of application • Site and length of application • Temperature of water • How the patient tolerated the procedure • The condition of the skin	___	___

Procedure Completed ________________________ **Date** ____________________

Notes ____

____

____

PROCEDURE

APPLYING DRY HEAT

Standard Precautions ☐ Handwashing ☐ Gloving ☐ Gowning ☐ Masking

Introductory Tasks ☐ Gather Equipment ☐ Identify/Introduce/Explain ☐ Provide Privacy

	Yes	No
5. Place a bath blanket over the patient. Make sure the parts of the body not being treated are covered.	___	___
6. Fanfold top linens down to the foot of the bed.	___	___
7. Uncover the part of the body that needs treatment.	___	___
8. Fill a pitcher with hot water. Using a bath thermometer, check the water temperature. It should be 115° F.	___	___
9. Pour the hot water into the water bottle. Stop when it is half full. Replace the cap, turning it tightly.	___	___
10. Lay the water bottle on a flat surface. To squeeze air out of the bottle, hold the neck of the bottle in an upright position. When you can see water in the neck of the bottle, the air has been squeezed out.	___	___

	Yes	No
11. Tighten the top on the bottle.	___	___
12. Check the bottle for leaks.	___	___
13. Dry the bottle if it has become wet.	___	___
14. Place the bottle in its flannel cover.	___	___
15. Place the bottle on the area needing heat treatment. Never place the bottle under the patient.	___	___
16. During treatment, check the area every 5 minutes for signs of blistering, swelling, or redness. Ask the patient if there is any pain, burning, or numbness. If there are any signs, remove the hot water bottle and report the problems to the nurse.	___	___
17. When the treatment is finished, remove the bottle.	___	___
18. Rearrange the top linens and remove the bath blanket.	___	___
19. Check to make sure the patient is comfortable and that the body is aligned properly.	___	___
20. Make sure the signal light is within the patient's reach.	___	___
21. Open the screen.	___	___
22. Clean the equipment and return it to storage.	___	___
23. Wash your hands.	___	___
24. Record your observations and report anything unusual to the nurse: • Time of application • Site and length of application • Temperature of water • How the patient tolerated the procedure • The condition of the skin	___	___

Procedure Completed ______________________ **Date** ______________

Notes ____

____

____

PROCEDURE

GIVING A WARM SOAK

Standard Precautions ☐ Handwashing ☐ Gloving ☐ Gowning ☐ Masking

Introductory Tasks ☐ Gather Equipment ☐ Identify/Introduce/Explain ☐ Provide Privacy

	Yes	No
5. Raise the bed to a comfortable working position.	___	___
6. Place a bath blanket over the patient. Make sure the parts of the body not being treated are covered.	___	___
7. Fanfold top linens down to the foot of the bed.	___	___
8. Uncover the part of the body that needs treatment.	___	___
9. Fill the basin half full with warm water. Using a bath thermometer, check the water temperature. It should be 105° to 110° F.	___	___
10. Position the waterproof mattress protector under the part of the body that will be soaked.	___	___
11. Position the basin so the part of the patient's body that needs treatment easily reaches the basin.	___	___
12. Gently lower the part being treated into the basin.	___	___
13. Monitor the temperature of the water in the basin every 5 minutes. When it loses its warmth, remove the patient's limb and wrap it in a towel. Repeat Steps 9, 11, and 12.	___	___
14. During treatment, check the area regularly for signs of blistering, swelling, or redness. Ask the patient if there is any pain, burning, or numbness. If there are any signs or symptoms, remove the limb from the basin and report the problems to the nurse.	___	___
15. When the treatment is finished, remove the basin and pat dry the treatment area.	___	___
16. Remove the mattress cover. Rearrange the top linens and remove the bath blanket.	___	___
17. Check to make sure the patient is comfortable and that the body is aligned properly.	___	___
18. Make sure the signal light is within the patient's reach.	___	___
19. Lower the bed.	___	___
20. Open the screen.	___	___
21. Clean the equipment and return it to storage.	___	___
22. Wash your hands.	___	___

	Yes	No
23. Record your observations and report anything unusual to the nurse: • Time procedure began and ended • Site that was soaked • How the patient tolerated the procedure • The condition of the skin	___	___

Procedure Completed ______________________ **Date** ______________________

Notes ______________________

____

____

PROCEDURE

GIVING A SITZ BATH

Standard Precautions ☐ Handwashing ☐ Gloving ☐ Gowning ☐ Masking

Introductory Tasks ☐ Gather Equipment ☐ Identify/Introduce/Explain ☐ Provide Privacy

	Yes	No
6. To prepare for the sitz bath, do one of the following: • If using a disposable sitz bath, position it on the toilet seat. • If using a portable sitz bath, position it alongside the patient's bed. • If using a built-in sitz bath, transport the patient by wheelchair to the room where the sitz bath is located.	___	___
7. Fill the sitz bath two-thirds full with water. The water temperature should be 105° F.	___	___
8. Place towels over metal parts of the sitz bath so no contact is made with the patient's skin. Also, place a towel on the seat and front edge of the bath.	___	___
9. Help the patient raise his or her gown and tie it loosely above the waist.	___	___
10. Assist the patient as he or she sits down on the sitz bath.	___	___
11. Cover the patient's legs and shoulders with bath blankets.	___	___
12. Make sure the patient is comfortable and that the signal light is within reach.	___	___
13. During the treatment, check the patient every 5 minutes. Ask about feeling weak, drowsy, or faint. If the patient says yes, call for a helper and return the patient to bed.	___	___
14. After 20 minutes, help the patient stand up. Assist with patting dry the patient and putting on a clean gown.	___	___
15. Help the patient get back in bed.	___	___
16. Check to make sure the patient is comfortable and that the body is aligned properly.	___	___

	Yes	No
17. Make sure the signal light is within the patient's reach.	___	___
18. Open the screen.	___	___
19. Using disinfectant solution, clean the sitz bath. Return reusable equipment to the proper location. Put used linens in the linen hamper.	___	___
20. Wash your hands.	___	___
21. Record your observations and report anything unusual to the nurse: • Time the procedure started and ended • Temperature of water • How the patient tolerated the procedure • The condition of the skin	___	___

Procedure Completed ______________________ **Date** ______________________

Notes ____

____

____

PROCEDURE

APPLYING A COLD PACK

Standard Precautions ☐ Handwashing ☐ Gloving ☐ Gowning ☐ Masking

Introductory Tasks ☐ Gather Equipment ☐ Identify/Introduce/Explain ☐ Provide Privacy

	Yes	No
6. Perform the action necessary to activate the cooling of the cold pack.	___	___
7. Place a flannel cover over the cold pack.	___	___
8. Place the covered cold pack over the site to be treated. Use ties, tape, or rolled gauze to hold the cold pack in place.	___	___
9. The cold pack can be left in place for up to 30 minutes. However, you must check the area every 10 minutes for skin discoloration and signs of blisters. Observe whether the patient is shivering or has signs of cyanosis. Ask the patient if there is any pain, burning, or numbness. If there are any signs, remove the cold pack and tell the nurse right away.	___	___
10. After 30 minutes, remove the tape (or ties or gauze), towel, and cold pack.	___	___
11. Check to make sure the patient is comfortable and that the body is aligned properly.	___	___
12. Make sure the signal light is within the patient's reach.	___	___

	Yes	No
13. Open the screen.	___	___
14. Wash your hands.	___	___
15. Record your observations and report anything unusual to the nurse: • Time the procedure started and ended • Site of application • How the patient tolerated the procedure • The condition of the skin	___	___

Procedure Completed ______________________ **Date** ______________

Notes ____

____

____

PROCEDURE

APPLYING A COLD COMPRESS

Standard Precautions ☐ Handwashing ☐ Gloving ☐ Gowning ☐ Masking

Introductory Tasks ☐ Gather Equipment ☐ Identify/Introduce/Explain ☐ Provide Privacy

	Yes	No
6. Fill the basin half full with cold water.	___	___
7. Put the compresses in the basin.	___	___
8. Place a bath blanket over the patient. Make sure the parts of the body not being treated are covered.	___	___
9. Fanfold top linens down to the foot of the bed.	___	___
10. Place a waterproof pad under the area being treated.	___	___
11. Uncover the part of the body that needs treatment.	___	___
12. Take a compress out of the basin and wring out the excess water.	___	___
13. Position the compress over the treatment area.	___	___
14. The cold compress can be left in place for up to 20 minutes. However, you must check the area every 5 minutes for skin discoloration and signs of blisters. Observe whether the patient is shivering or has signs of cyanosis. Ask the patient if there is any pain, burning, or numbness. If there are any signs, remove the cold pack and tell the nurse right away.	___	___
15. When the compress is no longer cold, replace it with another cold compress.	___	___

	Yes	No
16. After 20 minutes, remove the compress.	___	___
17. Using a towel, pat dry the skin where the compress was applied.	___	___
18. Check to make sure the patient is comfortable and that the body is aligned properly.	___	___
19. Make sure the signal light is within the patient's reach and the bed is in the low position.	___	___
20. Open the screen.	___	___
21. Clean the equipment and return it to storage.	___	___
22. Wash your hands.	___	___
23. Record your observations and report anything unusual to the nurse: • Time the procedure started and ended • Site of application • How the patient tolerated the procedure • The condition of the skin	___	___

Procedure Completed ______________________ **Date** ______________

Notes ____

____

____

PROCEDURE

GIVING A COLD SOAK

Standard Precautions ☐ Handwashing ☐ Gloving ☐ Gowning ☐ Masking

Introductory Tasks ☐ Gather Equipment ☐ Identify/Introduce/Explain ☐ Provide Privacy

	Yes	No
5. Place a bath blanket over the patient. Make sure the parts of the body not being treated are covered.	___	___
6. Fanfold top linens down to the foot of the bed.	___	___
7. Position the waterproof mattress protector under the part of the body that will be soaked.	___	___
8. Fill the basin half full with cold water.	___	___
9. Uncover the part of the body that needs treatment.	___	___
10. Position the basin so the part of the patient's body that needs treatment can easily reach the basin.	___	___
11. Gradually lower the part being treated into the basin.	___	___

	Yes	No
12. Monitor the temperature of the water in the basin every 5 minutes. When the water is no longer cold, remove the patient's limb and wrap it in a towel. Repeat Steps 8, 10, and 11.	___	___
13. During treatment, check the area every 5 minutes for skin discoloration and signs of blisters. Observe whether the patient is shivering or has signs of cyanosis. Ask the patient if there is any pain, burning, or numbness. If there are any signs, remove the limb from the basin and tell the nurse right away.	___	___
14. When treatment is finished, remove the basin. Pat dry the area.	___	___
15. Remove the mattress cover. Rearrange the top linens and remove the bath blanket.	___	___
16. Check to make sure the patient is comfortable and that the body is aligned properly.	___	___
17. Make sure the signal light is within the patient's reach.	___	___
18. Open the screen.	___	___
19. Clean the equipment and return it to storage.	___	___
20. Wash your hands.	___	___
21. Record your observations and report anything unusual to the nurse: • Time the procedure started and ended • Site of application • How the patient tolerated the procedure • The condition of the skin	___	___

Procedure Completed ______________________________ **Date** ____________________

Notes ____

____

____

PROCEDURE

GIVING A COLD BATH

Standard Precautions ☐ Handwashing ☐ Gloving ☐ Gowning ☐ Masking

Introductory Tasks ☐ Gather Equipment ☐ Identify/Introduce/Explain ☐ Provide Privacy

	Yes	No
6. Measure and record the patient's vital signs and the time.	___	___
7. Raise the bed to a comfortable working height. Lower the side rail (if applicable).	___	___
8. Place the bath blanket over the patient. Remove the top linens.	___	___
9. Remove the patient's gown. Take care not to expose the patient.	___	___

	Yes	No
10. Place ice bags or ice packs in covers.	___	___
11. Prepare the hot water bottle for use. Make sure it has a flannel cover on it.	___	___
12. With a helper, if necessary, move the patient to the side of the bed where you are working.	___	___
13. Position the ice bags or packs on the patient's forehead, under both armpits, and in the groin.	___	___
14. Place the hot water bottle on the patient's feet. (This helps prevent the patient from becoming excessively chilled.) Raise the side rail (if appropriate).	___	___
15. Fill the basin with cold water. Add alcohol, if ordered.	___	___
16. Place the washcloths in the basin. Lower the side rail (if appropriate).	___	___
17. Position a towel under the patient's arm on the far side of the bed.	___	___
18. Remove a washcloth from the basin. Wring out the excess water. Make sure there are no ice chips on the washcloth. Gently sponge the patient's arm for 5 minutes.	___	___
19. Using a towel, dry the arm by patting it gently; do not rub the skin.	___	___
20. Repeat Steps 18 and 19 for the other arm.	___	___
21. Measure and record the patient's vital signs and the time. If the body temperature is not within normal range, stop treatment.	___	___
22. Observe whether the patient is shivering or has signs of cyanosis. Ask the patient if there is any pain, burning, or numbness. If there are any signs, stop treatment and tell the nurse right away.	___	___
23. Put a towel under the patient's leg on the far side of the bed.	___	___
24. Take a washcloth from the basin, wring out the excess water, and gently sponge the leg for 5 minutes. Using a towel, pat the leg dry.	___	___
25. Repeat Steps 23 and 24 for the other leg.	___	___
26. Turn the patient so he or she is facing away from you. Get a helper, if necessary.	___	___
27. Put a towel on the mattress along the patient's back and buttocks.	___	___
28. Take a washcloth from the basin, wring out the excess water, and gently sponge the back and buttocks for 5 minutes. Pat the area dry with a towel.	___	___
29. Move the patient into the supine position (see Chapter 16). Make sure the patient is in the center of the bed.	___	___
30. Remove all ice bags and packs. Remove the hot water bottle.	___	___
31. Measure and record the patient's vital signs and the time.	___	___
32. Remove the bath blanket. Put a clean gown on the patient. As much as possible, avoid exposing the patient.	___	___
33. Check to see if the bed linens are wet or soiled. Change them, if necessary.	___	___
34. Check to make sure the patient is comfortable and that the body is aligned properly.	___	___
35. Make sure the signal light is within the patient's reach. Raise the side rail (if appropriate).	___	___
36. Open the screen.	___	___

	Yes	No
37. Clean the equipment and return it to storage.	___	___
38. Wash your hands.	___	___
39. Wait 30 minutes after the treatment; then return and measure the patient's vital signs.	___	___
40. Record your observations and report anything unusual to the nurse: • Time the procedure started and ended • Vital signs measurements • How the patient tolerated the procedure • The condition of the skin under hot and cold applications	___	___

Procedure Completed ______________________ **Date** ______________________

Notes ____

____

____

PROCEDURE

APPLYING A DRESSING

Standard Precautions ☐ Handwashing ☐ Gloving ☐ Gowning ☐ Masking

Introductory Tasks ☐ Gather Equipment ☐ Identify/Introduce/Explain ☐ Provide Privacy

	Yes	No
5. Place a paper towel on the over-bed table to provide a clean work area.	___	___
6. Open the waste container and place it within reach.	___	___
7. Cut pieces of tape for securing the dressing. For a 4 x 4 dressing, cut four pieces of 8-inch tape. Hang the cut tape from the over-bed table.	___	___
8. Open the package of 4 x 4 gauze. Do not touch the gauze. Lay the gauze package on the over-bed table.	___	___
9. Put on the gloves.	___	___
10. If there is an old dressing, remove it as follows: • Pull the tape toward the wound. • Lift the dressing off the wound. Pull off the dressing and remaining tape. You can hold the dressing with your gloved fingertips and pull off the glove over the dressing to contain the dressing for discarding. • Note the color of the wound and any drainage. • Place the old dressing and tape in a waste container. • Remove your gloves and place them in a waste container. • Put on clean gloves.	___	___

	Yes	No
11. Place the clean 4 x 4 gauze over the wound. Be careful to touch only the outer edges of the gauze.	___	___
12. Place tape over the edges of the gauze. Half the tape should be on the gauze and half on the skin.	___	___
13. Discard the gauze wrappers in a waste container.	___	___
14. Remove your gloves.	___	___
15. Wash your hands.	___	___
16. Report the following to the nurse: • Dressing was changed • Time of dressing change; wound condition • Any unusual observations	___	___

Procedure Completed ______________________ **Date** ______________________

Notes ____

____

____

PROCEDURE

APPLYING A BINDER

Standard Precautions ☐ Handwashing ☐ Gloving ☐ Gowning ☐ Masking

Introductory Tasks ☐ Gather Equipment ☐ Identify/Introduce/Explain ☐ Provide Privacy

	Yes	No
5. Help the resident turn toward you.	___	___
Follow these steps for a scultetus binder:		
6. Place the binder on the center of the bed. Put an edge of the binder under the resident's back.	___	___
7. Roll the resident onto his or her back. Pull the binder so it is centered behind the resident.	___	___
8. Close the binder by bringing each tail across the abdomen, starting at the bottom. Pull each strip taut and smooth.	___	___
9. Fasten the binder on top with Velcro. Always fasten according to the manufacturer's instructions. The binder should be snug but not too tight.	___	___
Follow this step for a T-binder:	___	___
10. Pull the strap between the resident's legs, covering the perineal dressings, and pin it to the waistband. Men use a modified T-binder.	___	___
11. Make the resident comfortable and provide for safety.	___	___

	Yes	No
13. Wash your hands.	___	___
14. Report the following to the nurse: • That you have applied the binder • How the resident tolerated the procedure • Any unusual observations	___	___

Procedure Completed ____________________ **Date** ____________________

Notes ____

____

____

PROCEDURE

APPLYING AN ELASTIC BANDAGE

Standard Precautions ☐ Handwashing ☐ Gloving ☐ Gowning ☐ Masking

Introductory Tasks ☐ Gather Equipment ☐ Identify/Introduce/Explain ☐ Provide Privacy

	Yes	No
5. Place the resident in a comfortable position.	___	___
6. Expose the area that is going to be wrapped.	___	___
7. Extend the body part to be bandaged. Support the resident's arm or leg.	___	___
8. Hold the bandage so the loose end is toward the resident.	___	___
9. Wrap the bandage two times around the limb to anchor it. Place the bandage on the narrowest part of the limb.	___	___
10. Wrap the bandage around the limb, toward the heart. Each spiral turn should overlap the previous one.	___	___
11. Make sure the bandage is smooth and secure, but not too tight.	___	___
12. Leave the fingers or toes exposed so you can inspect the skin.	___	___
13. After the bandage is completely wrapped, secure the end with the metal clips, Velcro, or tape.	___	___
14. If a second bandage is to be used, overlap it with the first.	___	___
15. Make the resident comfortable and provide for safety.	___	___
16. Open the screen.	___	___
17. Wash your hands.	___	___
18. Report the following to the nurse: • That you have applied the elastic bandage • The area where the bandage was applied • How the resident tolerated the procedure • Any unusual observations	___	___

Procedure Completed ______________________ **Date** ______________________

Notes ____

____

____

PROCEDURE

OBRA SP

PUTTING ON ELASTIC STOCKINGS

Standard Precautions ☐ Handwashing ☐ Gloving ☐ Gowning ☐ Masking

Introductory Tasks ☐ Gather Equipment ☐ Identify/Introduce/Explain ☐ Provide Privacy

	Yes	No
5. Make sure the elastic stockings are the correct size.	___	___
6. Raise the bed to a comfortable position and lower the side rail (if appropriate).	___	___
7. Have the resident lie on his or her back. Expose one leg by fanfolding the top covers to the bottom of the bed.	___	___
8. Hold the stocking with one hand and gather it so you are holding the foot of the stocking.	___	___
9. Place the foot of the stocking over the resident's toe and heel.	___	___
10. Roll the stocking up over the leg.	___	___
11. The stocking should be even along the leg. Make sure to smooth all creases and wrinkles.	___	___
12. Repeat the procedure on the other leg.	___	___
13. Cover the resident and make sure the resident is comfortable.	___	___
14. Provide for safety.	___	___

15. Open the screen.

16. Wash your hands.

17. Report the following to the nurse:
- The stockings have been applied
- The time the stockings were applied
- Any unusual observations

Procedure Completed ______________________ **Date** ______________________

Notes ____

____

____

CHAPTER 26

HOME HEALTH CARE

STUDY OBJECTIVES

Home health aides often train as nursing assistants. Jobs in home health care usually include communication with the client and family, personal record keeping, some housekeeping and food preparation, and reporting on the client's progress. Abuse in home health care has been widespread and is now being investigated in many states.

- Home health aides provide whatever personal care clients need. They also tend to housekeeping and food preparation duties. They usually do clients' laundry.
- Honesty, compassion, and independence are three important qualities needed for success in home health care work.
- Home health care aides communicate directly with clients during work or outside of work on the telephone. Most communication with client families, friends, and medical personnel is done on the telephone.
- Home health aides often have to keep daily reports indicating what work was done and when. Also, aides may need to keep expense records and mileage reports, as well as long-term reports.
- In emergencies, dial 911. Then, contact your supervisor, a doctor, or a family member to tell them about the emergency.
- A safe client care environment includes cleared pathways, a well-lit and well-ventilated room for the client, and, for clients who smoke, safe and frequently cleaned ashtrays.
- Housekeeping duties vary. Usually, the home health aide cleans up after food preparation and serving, handles the trash, does the laundry, and may do the bathroom. Sometimes, vacuuming, dusting, and floor washing may be included.
- Home health aides encourage independence by letting clients direct the management of their own households as much as possible. As soon as clients are able, they should be encouraged to handle as many of their own needs as they can.
- Home health aides usually report on clients' progress in written form. They may call family members to give verbal reports.
- Home health aides need to buy and serve food that meets nutritional and medical requirements and to respect cultural preferences as much as possible. Clients may need food that is cut fine or pureed.

- Clients may be physically abused. They may be psychologically threatened. Signs of abuse include a continuing pattern of bruises. Some clients may have been abandoned by family.

KNOW YOUR TERMS

In the space provided, write the letter of the definition that best fits the numbered term.

__ 1. abandonment	a. Care given by a substitute so as to give the primary caregiver a rest.
__ 2. home health assistant	b. Another name for home health assistant.
__ 3. home health care assistant	c. The withdrawal of needed support or help. In certain situations, may involve criminal liability.
__ 4. respite care	d. A person who works as a caregiver in home health care.

TEST YOUR KNOWLEDGE

Write the word(s) that best completes the statement.

1. Home health aides may be asked to help with ____________ chores.
2. Qualities important in home health care work are honesty, compassion, and ____________.
3. Agencies often require home health aides to fill out a daily ____________.
4. Dial ____________ in an emergency.
5. Keep all floor pathways ____________ so the client does not trip.
6. Most homes need ____________ once a week.
7. Counters used in ____________ ____________ should be cleaned as soon as possible.
8. The ____________ label on food packages tells you the amounts of fats, carbohydrates, and proteins in each serving of that food.
9. Helping the client regain movement is a way to promote ____________.
10. ____________ is being left without support or care.

THINK ABOUT THE ISSUES

1. A client wants to do more than she seems physically capable of doing. How should you handle this situation, making sure to prevent the client from getting hurt?
2. Some elderly are abandoned by family who cannot take care of them. Do you think they should be held accountable? Why or why not?

▲ CHECK YOUR SKILLS

In the following procedure checklists, check each task box that applies and answer yes or no to each step you have completed. If possible, have your instructor sign off when you have completed a procedure.

PROCEDURE

CHECKING A FOOD LABEL

	Yes	No
1. Examine the client's dietary restriction list and note the specific restrictions.	___	___
2. Look at the food label and find any items that are on the restriction list.	___	___
3. Compare the amount of the restricted item permitted to the amount indicated in a serving. For example, the diabetic exchanges allowed should be compared to the number on the label.	___	___
4. If the amount of the restricted item is acceptable, you may give the food to the client.	___	___
5. If the amount is not acceptable, mark the can as not to be used. Do not purchase the item if you are shopping for the client.	___	___

Procedure Completed______________________________ **Date**____________________

Notes____

CHAPTER 27

UNDERSTANDING MENTAL HEALTH

STUDY OBJECTIVES

Mental health is often affected by chronic illness and the effects of aging. Alzheimer's disease is a mental disorder that affects mostly elderly people. The elderly also have a high proportion of people with depression, schizophrenia, and various other types of dementia.

▲ Some major mental disorders that afflict people in long-term care are schizophrenia and Alzheimer's disease.

▲ People with Alzheimer's disease gradually lose mental functioning. This leads to safety problems, wandering, forgetfulness, and eventually loss of physical functioning.

▲ Never be confrontational to patients with schizophrenia. Encourage them to stay calm and take their medication.

▲ People with depression may become suicidal. They may also not communicate, not take care of themselves, and not eat.

▲ Delirium, disorientation, and confusion may be caused by illness, excessive alcohol intake, a reaction to medication, a high fever, or a traumatic injury.

▲ Being patient and understanding helps patients with dementia. Reality orientation may improve memory and understanding.

▲ People with severe anxiety may be helped by talk therapy or medication.

KNOW YOUR TERMS

In the space provided, write the letter of the definition that best fits the numbered term.

__ 1. agitation	a. A state of well-being of the mind and emotions.
__ 2. alcoholism	b. A severe mental disorder in which the person's thought process is defective.
__ 3. anxiety	c. A state of mental disturbance characterized by mixing things up.
__ 4. confusion	d. A false belief in one's ill health.
__ 5. delirium	e. A severe mental disorder characterized by feelings of persecution.
__ 6. delusion	f. A behavior characteristic of Alzheimer's disease in which patients become agitated toward the end of the day.
__ 7. dementia	g. A false perception of reality arising from a mental disorder.
__ 8. hallucination	h. A psychotic, usually persistent, thought present in some mental illnesses.
__ 9. hypochondria	i. A common form of psychosis characterized by irrational and illogical thoughts and the hearing of inner voices.
__10. mental health	j. A deteriorated mental state; madness.
__11. paranoia	k. A feeling of dread without a specific reason.
__12. psychosis	l. State of mind characterized by disturbed and overly excited feelings.
__13. schizophrenia	m. A disease characterized by chronic dependence on or abuse of alcohol.
__14. sundowning	n. A mental disturbance usually caused by a physical condition and often characterized by unintelligible speech, extreme agitation, or hallucinations.

TEST YOUR KNOWLEDGE

Write the word(s) that best completes the statement.

1. ____________ is the level of natural growth and development appropriate to a specific age group.
2. ____________ disease is a common dementia among the elderly.
3. Behavior change at dusk is called ____________
4. Stage ____________ is the most severe stage of Alzheimer's disease.
5. The general term for any severe disorder in which the mental state is defective is ____________.

6. Patients with _____________ typically hear inner voices.
7. One treatment for alcoholism involves complete _____________.
8. _____________ is a feeling of dread without a specific reason.
9. _____________ is a state of extreme restlessness.
10. _____________ are false perceptions of reality.

THINK ABOUT THE ISSUES

1. Some people with mental disorders are very insistent about their view of reality. How do you think you would feel working with such people?
2. Alzheimer's disease has no cure. How would you deal with a family member with Stage 3 Alzheimer's disease?

CHAPTER 28

CARING FOR THE NEWBORN

STUDY OBJECTIVES

Newborns require care from the moment they are born. Knowing the signs of newborn illness, how to hold a baby, and how to assist the new mother in feeding, burping, bathing, and changing are all essential to nursing assistants who help care for newborns.

- The basic steps in newborn care are preparing formula, feeding, burping, diapering, bathing, and providing circumcision and umbilical cord care as necessary.
- Signs of illness in newborns are high fever, unusual breathing patterns and sounds, abnormal stools, unusual restlessness or limpness, vomiting, excessive crying, swelling, rash, coughing, and refusing to eat.
- To bottle-feed a baby, prepare the formula, warm the bottle, find a quiet, comfortable spot, feed and burp the baby.
- To change a diaper, gather all needed supplies, remove the soiled diaper, clean the newborn, put on a clean diaper, and dress.
- To care for the umbilical cord, wipe clean with a cotton ball dipped in alcohol. Umbilical cord care is done during a diaper change.
- To provide circumcision care, wipe the perineal area clean; then apply petroleum jelly to the circumcision site with a gauze pad or cotton swab.
- Set up the bath in a safe container with the bathwater at an appropriately warm temperature. Hold the baby firmly and wash the eyes, then the head and body, and lastly, the perineal area.
- To burp an infant, hold the infant upright and rub or pat the back gently until the air is released.
- To weigh an infant, place a disposable pad on the scale, set the level to zero, place the undressed infant on the scale, and take the measurement.
- Safety concerns in the infant's environment include making sure all hot or dangerous items are kept out of reach, putting the baby to sleep on its back, holding the baby securely, and never leaving the baby unattended in a dangerous spot.

KNOW YOUR TERMS

In the space provided, write the letter of the definition that best fits the numbered term.

__ 1. bonding	a. An operation to remove some or all of the prepuce.
__ 2. bottle-feed	b. Breast milk secreted for the first few days after birth.
__ 3. breast-feed	c. To feed an infant by suckling at the mother's breasts.
__ 4. circumcision	d. The formation of a close relationship, as between a mother and a newborn.
__ 5. colostrum	e. To feed infants by bottle.
__ 6. fontanel	f. In a health care facility, the sharing of a room by mother and child after birth.
__ 7. nurse (v.)	g. To wrap an infant tightly in a cloth that restricts movement.
__ 8. rooming-in	h. A reflex that causes infants to search around for something to suck.
__ 9. rooting reflex	i. A cord that goes from the navel of a fetus to the placenta and through which the fetus receives nourishment.
__10. swaddle	j. A membrane-covered opening in the skull of an infant.
__11. umbilical cord	k. To feed an infant from a mother's breast.

TEST YOUR KNOWLEDGE

Write the word(s) that best completes the statement.

1. ____________ is the process of mother and infant getting to know each other.
2. The soft spots at the top of a newborn's head are called ____________.
3. Fever over ____________ is a sign of newborn illness.
4. Babies are sometimes wrapped or ____________ in a receiving blanket.
5. The thick yellow fluid that is fed to breast-fed babies in the first few days is the ____________.
6. The ____________ reflex causes babies to look for something to suck.
7. The ____________ ____________ connects the baby to the mother's placenta.
8. ____________ care should be given every time the diaper is changed.
9. Babies need to ____________ to release air from their stomachs.
10. Babies should always sleep on their ____________.

▲ THINK ABOUT THE ISSUES

1. If an infant refuses to eat, what should you do?
2. Some infants cry constantly. What are some of the ways to comfort infants?

▲ CHECK YOUR SKILLS

In the following procedure checklists, check each task box that applies and answer yes or no to each step you have completed. If possible, have your instructor sign off when you have completed a procedure.

PROCEDURE

SP

BOTTLE-FEEDING AN INFANT

Standard Precautions ☐ Handwashing ☐ Gloving ☐ Gowning ☐ Masking

Introductory Tasks ☐ Gather Equipment ☐ Identify/Introduce/Explain ☐ Provide Privacy

	Yes	No
4. Check the temperature of the formula.	___	___
5. Sit in a comfortable chair holding the infant. Support the infant's head and shoulders in your arm. Place the bib under the baby's chin.	___	___
6. Tilt the bottle and place the nipple in the infant's mouth. Keep the bottle upright so the nipple and neck remain filled with formula.	___	___
7. Let the infant drink at its own pace.	___	___
8. Look at the infant and speak gently.	___	___
9. About halfway through the feeding, burp the baby (see Burping a Newborn).	___	___
10. Continue feeding and burping until the infant either finishes the bottle or stops sucking.	___	___
11. Clean the baby's face and neck.	___	___
12. Place the infant in the bassinet. Do not use a pillow.	___	___
13. Discard extra formula. Discard disposable feeding supplies.	___	___
14. Record the time of the feeding and the amount consumed.	___	___
15. Put the laundry in the hamper.	___	___
16. Wash out reusable feeding supplies.	___	___
17. Wash your hands.	___	___

Procedure Completed ______________________ **Date** ______________________

Notes ____

____

____

PROCEDURE

CHANGING AN INFANT'S DIAPER

Standard Precautions ☐ Handwashing ☐ Gloving ☐ Gowning ☐ Masking

Introductory Tasks ☐ Gather Equipment ☐ Identify/Introduce/Explain ☐ Provide Privacy

	Yes	No
4. Place the changing pad on the changing table in the nursery or under the baby in the bassinet in the mother's room.	___	___
5. Put on your gloves.	___	___
6. Loosen the soiled diaper. Bring the front piece down between the legs.	___	___
7. Use the front of the diaper to wipe feces off the baby's genitals and buttocks. Wipe from front to back.	___	___
8. Hold the baby's ankles and lift the buttocks.	___	___
9. Place the soiled diaper in a disposable bag or diaper pail.	___	___
10. Dip a cotton ball in water and clean the baby's perineal area. Wipe from front to back with a clean cotton ball for each swab.	___	___
11. Use more wet cotton balls until the baby is clean.	___	___
12. Open the clean diaper and place it under the baby's buttocks.	___	___
13. Apply any creams or ointments necessary. Pediatricians may prescribe ointments or, in a home situation, the mother and father may have preferences.	___	___
14. Pull the loose part up between the legs and adjust so the diaper fits snugly. A cloth diaper is arranged so that the extra fold is in the front for boys and in the back for girls. Gently point a boy's penis downward so that urine does not go up out of the diaper. If a circumcision has not healed, make sure the diaper is loose in that area. Also, if the cord stump has not healed, position the diaper below the navel.	___	___
15. Fasten the diaper using the adhesive strips or the diaper pins or diaper cover. Fasten diaper pins so they point away from the abdomen.	___	___
16. Place the baby back in the bassinet or crib. Make sure the baby is safe and comfortable.	___	___

	Yes	No
17. Remove your equipment.	___	___
18. Empty soiled diapers, if necessary. Discard the disposable pad, used cotton balls, and soiled diaper, if not already done. Rinse cloth diapers before placing them in a covered container.	___	___
19. Remove your gloves.	___	___
20. Wash your hands.	___	___

21. Report and record the following:
- Time of diaper change
- Amount and color of urine or feces
- Ointments or creams used
- Condition of skin

Procedure Completed ______________________ **Date** ______________________

Notes ____

____

____

PROCEDURE

CARING FOR AN UMBILICAL CORD

Standard Precautions ☐ Handwashing ☐ Gloving ☐ Gowning ☐ Masking

Introductory Tasks ☐ Gather Equipment ☐ Identify/Introduce/Explain ☐ Provide Privacy

	Yes	No
7. Follow Procedure, Changing an Infant's Diaper.	___	___
8. After you have cleaned the baby's perineal area, open the clean diaper and place it under the baby's buttocks.	___	___
9. Dip a cotton ball in alcohol and use it to wipe the base of the umbilical stump.	___	___
10. Finish diapering the baby. Make sure you fold down the front of the diaper so it does not interfere with the umbilical stump.	___	___
11. Place the baby back in the bassinet or crib and make sure the baby is safe and comfortable.	___	___
12. Remove your equipment.	___	___
13. Empty soiled diaper, if necessary. Discard the disposable pad, used cotton balls, and soiled diaper. Rinse any soiled cloth diapers.	___	___

	Yes	No
14. Remove your gloves.	___	___
15. Wash your hands.	___	___
16. Report and record the following: • Time of diaper change • Amount and color of urine or feces • Umbilical cord care that was provided • Condition of the umbilical stump	___	___

Procedure Completed ______________________ **Date** ______________________

Notes ____

____

____

PROCEDURE

SP

CARING FOR A CIRCUMCISED BABY

Standard Precautions ☐ Handwashing ☐ Gloving ☐ Gowning ☐ Masking

Introductory Tasks ☐ Gather Equipment ☐ Identify/Introduce/Explain ☐ Provide Privacy

	Yes	No
7. Follow Procedure, Changing an Infant's Diaper.	___	___
8. After you have cleaned the baby's perineal area, open the clean diaper and place it under the baby's buttocks.	___	___
9. Put a generous amount of petroleum jelly on a gauze pad or cotton swab. Gently apply it to the penis. (Some facilities apply a lubricated gauze.)	___	___
10. Finish diapering the baby.	___	___
11. Place the baby back in the bassinet or crib. Make the baby comfortable and provide for safety.	___	___
12. Remove your equipment.	___	___
13. Empty soiled diaper, if necessary. Discard the disposable pad, used cotton balls, and soiled diaper. Rinse the soiled cloth diaper before placing it in a covered container.	___	___
14. Remove your gloves.	___	___
15. Wash your hands.	___	___

	Yes	No
16. Report and record the following: • Time of diaper change • Amount and color of urine or feces • Circumcision care that was provided • Condition of skin around the circumcision	___	___

Procedure Completed ______________________ **Date** ______________

Notes ____

____

____

PROCEDURE

BATHING A NEWBORN

Standard Precautions ☐ Handwashing ☐ Gloving ☐ Gowning ☐ Masking

Introductory Tasks ☐ Gather Equipment ☐ Identify/Introduce/Explain ☐ Provide Privacy

	Yes	No
3. Fill the washbasin with warm water. The water should be between 90° and 100° F. If you are testing the water by touching it with the inside of your wrist, it should feel warm and comfortable.	___	___
4. Support the baby. Wash the baby's eyes by dipping a cotton ball in water. Squeeze out the water.	___	___
5. Clean one eye from the inner to the outer corner. Clean the other eye with a clean cotton ball.	___	___
6. With another cotton ball, wipe around the ears and neck to clean away dried sweat.	___	___
7. With a clean cottonball, clean around the mouth and chin creases.	___	___
8. Dampen a clean washcloth with water. Wipe the hands and check for sharp fingernails.	___	___
9. Take off the diaper. *Note:* If you are working in a hospital, you may be required to put gloves on now. At home, it is wise to wear gloves or to put plastic baggies on your hands. Remember: Never leave the baby unattended.	___	___
10. Put soap on the washcloth and wash the baby's buttocks and perineal area. A male baby's scrotum may wrinkle up from the cool air or water.	___	___
11. Rinse with a clean washcloth and pat dry. Dry between folds of skin.	___	___

	Yes	No
12. Provide care to the umbilical stump and circumcision (males).	___	___
13. Apply lotions and powders as prescribed by the pediatrician or preferred by the parents.	___	___
14. Diaper the baby. Dress the baby in clean clothes.	___	___
15. Swaddle the baby in a receiving blanket.	___	___
16. Place the baby back in the bassinet and make sure it is safe and comfortable.	___	___
17. Clean the bath supplies and store them for the next use.	___	___
18. Clean the bath area. Remove your gloves.	___	___
19. Wash your hands.	___	___
20. Record the time of the bath.	___	___
21. Report any unusual observations (rashes, blood, bruising) to the nurse.	___	___

Procedure Completed ______________________ **Date** ______________________

Notes ____

____

____

PROCEDURE

WEIGHING A NEWBORN

Standard Precautions ☐ Handwashing ☐ Gloving ☐ Gowning ☐ Masking

Introductory Tasks ☐ Gather Equipment ☐ Identify/Introduce/Explain ☐ Provide Privacy

	Yes	No
3. Carry the baby to the room with the scale.	___	___
4. Undress the baby on the changing table. Remove all clothing, including the diaper.	___	___
5. Clean the baby's perineal area, if necessary.	___	___
6. Wrap the baby in a receiving blanket to keep it warm, until you place it on the scale.	___	___
7. Place the disposable pad on the scale and level the scale to zero.	___	___
8. Place the baby on its back on the scale.	___	___
9. Most infant scales have beveled sides to prevent the baby from slipping off. Other scales have a safety belt, which you should fasten. Keep one hand over the baby to prevent it from falling.	___	___

	Yes	No
10. Move the pointer of the pound calculation until it is almost level. Adjust the ounces calculation until the scale is level.	___	___
11. Record the weight and slide the pointers back to zero with one hand. Hold onto the baby with the other.	___	___
12. Lift the baby from the scale and wrap it in the blanket.	___	___
13. Remove the pad and discard it.	___	___
14. Diaper and dress the baby.	___	___
15. Return the baby to the bassinet or crib. Make sure the baby is safe and comfortable.	___	___
16. Wash your hands.	___	___
17. Record the time, date, and weight on the baby's chart.	___	___

Procedure Completed ______________________________ **Date** ______________________

Notes ____

____

____

CHAPTER 29

CARING FOR THE POSTPARTUM PATIENT

STUDY OBJECTIVES

The postpartum patient needs help in caring for the baby and in getting enough rest. Nursing assistants may help clean the home, care for the newborn, help the mother breast-feed, and help with older children.

- While still in the hospital, the postpartum patient may need help getting to the toilet and may also need help with perineal care.
- In a home setting, nursing assistants can help new mothers by caring for the home, older children, and the newborn as requested by the mother.
- To help the new mother breast-feed, bring the mother a beverage, set her up in a comfortable position, help her position the baby, and encourage her to get the baby started at the nipple.

KNOW YOUR TERMS

In the space provided, write the letter of the definition that best fits the numbered term.

__ 1. episiotomy	a. The release of breast milk in response to the presence of milk in the breast.
__ 2. letdown reflex	b. The normal blood that flows for a short time after childbirth.
__ 3. lochia	c. Surgical cutting of the vulva at the time of birth to avoid tearing.

TEST YOUR KNOWLEDGE

Write the word(s) that best completes the statement.

1. A small cut made in the perineum during the birth of a baby is called an ____________.
2. A serious mental disorder after birth is called ____________ ____________.
3. The area around the breast nipple is called the ____________.
4. The mother should nurse the baby on one breast for no more than ____________ minutes.
5. The mother's breasts release milk in response to the ____________ ____________.
6. The nursing mother needs ____________ extra calories per day to produce enough milk.
7. ____________ breasts are swollen and painful.
8. Pumping breast milk out by hand is called ____________ milk.
9. After nursing, always ____________ the baby.
10. Coffee and chocolate eaten by the mother may ____________ or ____________ the baby.

THINK ABOUT THE ISSUES

1. Some new mothers find breast-feeding difficult at first. What are some of the ways to encourage them to breast-feed?
2. If you suspect that the new mother has postpartum depression, what should you do?

CHECK YOUR SKILLS

In the following procedure checklists, check each task box that applies and answer yes or no to each step you have completed. If possible, have your instructor sign off when you have completed a procedure.

PROCEDURE

HELPING A NEW MOTHER BREAST-FEED

Standard Precautions ☐ Handwashing ☐ Gloving ☐ Gowning ☐ Masking

Introductory Tasks ☐ Gather Equipment ☐ Identify/Introduce/Explain ☐ Provide Privacy

Step	Yes	No
4. Assist the mother into a comfortable position. This can be sitting in a chair or lying in bed on her side.	___	___
5. Assist the mother in washing her hands.	___	___
6. If the mother is sitting in a chair, offer her a pillow to support the baby on her lap.	___	___
7. Hand the mother her baby.	___	___
8. Help position the baby so both mother and child are comfortable.	___	___
9. The mother should support the baby with one arm and support her breast with the other hand.	___	___
10. The mother should grasp her breast just above the areola.	___	___
11. Instruct the mother to brush the baby's cheek closest to the breast with the nipple. The baby will turn toward the nipple with his or her mouth open.	___	___
12. The mother gently places her nipple into the baby's mouth so the baby can latch on.	___	___
13. If this is temporarily painful for the mother, encourage her to relax.	___	___
14. Make sure the baby has taken hold of the nipple and areola.	___	___
15. Instruct the mother to use her thumb or finger to hold her breast away from the baby's nose so the baby can breathe properly.	___	___
16. Watch the baby's cheek for signs of sucking and swallowing.	___	___
17. The mother should nurse on the first breast for no more than 10 minutes.	___	___
18. Teach the mother to break the baby's suction by placing her forefinger between the areola and the baby's mouth.	___	___
19. Help the mother burp the baby (if she asks; if not, encourage her to do it after the baby finishes feeding at each breast).	___	___
20. The mother then nurses the baby on the second breast until the baby falls asleep or loses interest.	___	___
21. Burp the baby again.	___	___
22. The mother may ask you to change the baby's diaper or to help settle the baby in the bassinet.	___	___

	Yes	No
23. Help the mother wash the nipple and areola with a clean cotton ball moistened with warm water only (no soap). The mother should pat the nipple dry and allow it to air dry completely.	___	___
24. Help the mother put a tissue or safety pin on the bra strap of the breast she finished to remind her to begin on that side for the next feeding.	___	___
25. Give the mother fresh pads for her bra.	___	___
26. Assist the mother into a comfortable position.	___	___
27. Wash your hands.	___	___

Procedure Completed ______________________ **Date** ______________________

Notes ____

____

____

CHAPTER 30

CARING FOR THE TERMINALLY ILL

STUDY OBJECTIVES

Nursing assistants care for patients who are terminally ill by providing the same personal care as they would to all patients, encouraging such patients to express themselves as they wish, and helping them remain as comfortable as possible.

- Some people have a greater need for spiritual faith during a terminal illness. They may wish to have clergy visit them or they may wish for private time to examine their own spirituality.
- Patients who are terminally ill usually need help with personal care, particularly care of the nose and mouth and elimination needs. Feeding should be according to instructions in the patient's chart.
- Nursing assistants can help patients' families by providing privacy during visits, listening to their concerns, assisting them as much as possible, and being sensitive to their emotional needs.

KNOW YOUR TERMS

Define terminal illness:

____

____

TEST YOUR KNOWLEDGE

Write the word(s) that best completes the statement.

1. A ______________ illness is one in which there is no hope of recovery.
2. ______________ provide supportive comfortable care for patients who are terminally ill.
3. Patients with breathing problems usually find ______________-______________ position most comfortable.
4. Some terminally ill patients lose ______________ and/or ______________ control.
5. Patients near death often have ______________ appetites.
6. Some patients secrete ______________ into the mouth.
7. All dying patients have ______________ needs.
8. Do not give ______________ hope to a dying patient.
9. One way to comfort a dying patient is with a ______________ touch.
10. Many patients with ______________ choose hospice care.

THINK ABOUT THE ISSUES

1. Working with people who are dying makes you face your own feelings about death. Do you think you would be comfortable working with such patients? Why or why not?
2. What are some of the ways to communicate with patients who are terminally ill?

CHAPTER 31

DEATH AND POSTMORTEM CARE

STUDY OBJECTIVES

There are stages of dying that most patients go through. The typical signs of approaching death are slowed circulation and respiration, loss of muscle control, and changes in mental state and senses. Nursing assistants provide postmortem care according to facility policy.

- ▲ The stages of dying are denial, anger, bargaining, depression, and acceptance.
- ▲ The typical signs of approaching death are slowed circulation and respiration, loss of muscle control, and changes in mental state and senses.
- ▲ The four indications of death are no pulse, no respiration, no blood pressure, and fixed and dilated eyes.
- ▲ After death, the nursing assistant follows facility policy to clean and shroud the body.

KNOW YOUR TERMS

In the space provided, write the letter of the definition that best fits the numbered term.

__ 1. Cheyne-Stokes respiration	a. A cloth used to cover a dead body.
__ 2. DNR	b. A place where dead bodies are kept until identified and removed for burial.
__ 3. expire	c. An order that means the same as DNR.
__ 4. morgue	d. After death.
__ 5. no-code order	e. An order meaning Do Not Resuscitate, put on the chart of patients who are near death and who have chosen or whose proxy has chosen to allow natural death without extraordinary medical intervention.
__ 6. postmortem	f. To die.
__ 7. rigor mortis	g. An irregular breathing pattern with deep inhalation followed by apnea, characteristic of patients in a coma.
__ 8. shroud	h. A stiffening of the body after death.

TEST YOUR KNOWLEDGE

Write the word(s) that best completes the statement.

1. _____________ is the stage at which patients refuse to accept that death is impending.
2. _____________ is the stage at which patients express their rage.
3. _____________ is the stage at which patients try to arrange for more time to live.
4. _____________ is the stage at which patients realize they cannot change the outcome.
5. _____________ is the final stage at which patients begin to say good-bye.
6. _____________-_____________ respirations are a sign of impending death.
7. DNR means _____________ _____________ _____________.
8. No pulse, no respiration, and no blood pressure are all signs of _____________.
9. _____________ _____________ is a condition in which the body begins to stiffen after death.
10. _____________ care includes cleaning and putting a shroud on the body.

THINK ABOUT THE ISSUES

1. Have you ever seen or touched a dead body? Do you think you will be able to provide postmortem care?
2. Will you be able to honor a DNR order and let a patient die without trying to revive him or her?

CHECK YOUR SKILLS

In the following procedure checklists, check each task box that applies and answer yes or no to each step you have completed. If possible, have your instructor sign off when you have completed a procedure.

PROCEDURE

OBRA SP

GIVING POSTMORTEM CARE

Standard Precautions ☐ Handwashing ☐ Gloving ☐ Gowning ☐ Masking

Introductory Tasks ☐ Gather Equipment ☐ Identify/Introduce/Explain ☐ Provide Privacy

	Yes	No
3. Raise the bed to the highest comfortable level for working and make sure the bed is flat.	___	___
4. Put on gloves.	___	___
5. Position the body on its back, and elevate the head and shoulders on a pillow.	___	___
6. Close the eyes. Put a moistened cotton ball on each eyelid if the eyes do not stay closed.	___	___
7. Replace dentures or artificial eyes, unless otherwise instructed.	___	___
8. Close the mouth and, if necessary, gently support the jaw with a light bandage or a rolled hand towel.	___	___
9. If instructed, remove drainage bags, bottles, and containers. After checking with the nurse, remove tubes or catheters. The policy on removal of these items varies, so make sure you have permission.	___	___
10. Remove and list jewelry except engagement and wedding rings (check the facility's procedure).	___	___
11. Bathe and dry soiled areas as needed.	___	___
12. Place a bed protector under the buttocks and put on clean dressings.	___	___
13. Groom hair.	___	___
14. Fill out the identification tags and attach one to the right ankle or right big toe.	___	___
15. Cover the body up to the shoulders if the family will view it.	___	___
16. Gather all possessions in a labeled bag.	___	___
17. Remove all equipment and supplies except the shroud and tags. Make sure the room is neat and softly lit.	___	___
18. Provide privacy while the body is viewed. Give the family the person's possessions.	___	___

	Yes	No
19. Get a stretcher.	___	___
20. Follow the procedures of the facility. Generally, you place the body on the shroud and apply it as follows: • Bring the top down over the head. • Fold the bottom up over the feet. • Fold the sides over the body and secure the shroud.	___	___
21. Apply an identification tag to the shroud.	___	___
22. With assistance from other workers, move the body to the stretcher.	___	___
23. If appropriate, transport the body to the morgue. Make sure the doors to other patient rooms along the hallway are closed.	___	___
24. Return the stretcher to its proper location.	___	___
25. Remove all linens and supplies from the patient's room.	___	___
26. Remove the gloves and wash your hands.	___	___
27. Report the following to the nurse: • The time the body was transported • What was done with all personal belongings	___	___

Procedure Completed ______________________ **Date** ______________________

Notes ____

____

____

Answer Key

Chapter 1

▲ KNOW YOUR TERMS

1. o
2. u
3. h
4. e
5. w
6. m
7. l
8. g
9. t
10. p
11. i
12. s.
13. j
14. d
15. n
16. a
17. c
18. q
19. r
20. k
21. v
22. b
23. f

▲ TEST YOUR KNOWLEDGE

1. honesty, dependability, conscientiousness, empathy, patience, helpfulness, professionalism, objectivity, and a positive attitude. Any two of the preceding are correct.
2. conscientious
3. patient
4. nursing assistant
5. medication
6. diagnose
7. OBRA
8. infection
9. home health aide
10. increasing

Chapter 2

▲ KNOW YOUR TERMS

1. e
2. d
3. l
4. j
5. k
6. b
7. p
8. n
9. c
10. a
11. t
12. s
13. h
14. o
15. g
16. q
17. r
18. m
19. i
20. f

▲ TEST YOUR KNOWLEDGE

1. subacute
2. nursing home, skilled
3. adult day-care center
4. terminally ill
5. hospital
6. housekeeping
7. preferred provider organization
8. health maintenance organizations
9. 65
10. poor

CHAPTER 3

▲ KNOW YOUR TERMS

MATCHING EXERCISE I

1. d
2. g
3. m
4. l
5. f
6. j
7. a
8. i
9. b
10. k
11. e
12. n
13. c
14. h

MATCHING EXERCISE II

1. c
2. i
3. h
4. f
5. m
6. k
7. d
8. e
9. l
10. b
11. a
12. j
13. g

▲ TEST YOUR KNOWLEDGE

1. privacy
2. ombudsman
3. legal
4. ethical
5. nonverbal
6. active
7. closed-ended
8. open-ended
9. health care proxy
10. call signal

CHAPTER 4

▲ KNOW YOUR TERMS

1. f
2. r
3. l
4. g
5. a
6. h
7. b
8. e
9. d
10. n
11. j
12. c
13. s
14. i
15. k
16. o
17. t
18. p
19. m
20. q

▲ TEST YOUR KNOWLEDGE

1. air, water, food
2. Social
3. chronic
4. acute
5. Geriatric
6. Alzheimer's
7. independent
8. postpartum
9. culture
10. families

Chapter 5

▲ Know Your Terms

1. g
2. s
3. e
4. a
5. o
6. b
7. p
8. m
9. c
10. q
11. j
12. h
13. d
14. k
15. f
16. n
17. i
18. l
19. r

▲ Test Your Knowledge

1. neonate
2. 3, 5
3. primary period
4. puberty
5. peer pressure
6. Adolescence
7. young adulthood
8. menopause
9. late adulthood
10. personality

Chapter 6

▲ Know Your Terms

1. e
2. c
3. f
4. a
5. b
6. o
7. q
8. n
9. j
10. t
11. r
12. g
13. d
14. k
15. p
16. h
17. m
18. i
19. l
20. s

▲ Test Your Knowledge

1. emergency
2. remove patients
3. heatstroke
4. restraint
5. oxygen
6. standard precautions
7. handwashing
8. gloves
9. gown, mask
10. nonskid

Chapter 7

▲ KNOW YOUR TERMS

1. i
2. o
3. g
4. a
5. s
6. e
7. d
8. n
9. c
10. l
11. t
12. h
13. b
14. f
15. q
16. j
17. m
18. p
19. k
20. u
21. r

▲ TEST YOUR KNOWLEDGE

1. respiratory arrest
2. Cardiac arrest
3. Cardiopulmonary resuscitation
4. Heimlich maneuver
5. higher
6. stroke
7. pressure
8. tonic-clonic, generalized absence
9. second- or third-, first-
10. toxin

Chapter 8

▲ KNOW YOUR TERMS

1. f
2. c
3. a
4. d
5. b
6. e

▲ TEST YOUR KNOWLEDGE

1. client
2. classified ads
3. agencies
4. personal data sheet
5. job interview
6. reference
7. Cleanliness, neatness
8. clearly
9. letter
10. job search

Chapter 9

▲ KNOW YOUR TERMS

MATCHING EXERCISE I

1. k
2. m
3. o
4. r
5. l
6. a
7. n
8. d
9. j
10. e
11. h
12. c
13. b
14. f
15. q
16. g
17. i
18. p

MATCHING EXERCISE II

1. i
2. a
3. l
4. k
5. o
6. b
7. r
8. q
9. e
10. c
11. d
12. g
13. n
14. j
15. m
16. f
17. p
18. h

▲ TEST YOUR KNOWLEDGE

1. cell
2. Tissues
3. Organs
4. brain
5. eyes, ear, nose, skin, taste buds
6. decreases
7. low-pitched, high-pitched
8. skin
9. masturbation
10. Bisexuality

CHAPTER 10

KNOW YOUR TERMS

MATCHING EXERCISE I

1. m
2. z
3. j
4. o
5. s
6. k
7. a
8. b
9. w
10. c
11. v
12. y
13. g
14. p
15. t
16. x
17. u
18. i
19. f
20. d
21. r
22. e
23. l
24. h
25. n
26. q

MATCHING EXERCISE II

1. s
2. j
3. k
4. h
5. z
6. a
7. i
8. d
9. b
10. p
11. c
12. q
13. f
14. x
15. u
16. e
17. n
18. l
19. g
20. r
21. m
22. o
23. t
24. v
25. y
26. w

MATCHING EXERCISE III

1. k
2. d
3. h
4. a
5. g
6. b
7. c
8. f
9. e
10. p
11. m
12. i
13. j
14. l
15. n
16. o

TEST YOUR KNOWLEDGE

1. membrane, cytoplasm, nucleus
2. females
3. Connective
4. Epithelial
5. dorsal
6. ventral
7. circulatory system
8. urinary system
9. voluntary and involuntary
10. integumentary system

Chapter 11

▲ KNOW YOUR TERMS

MATCHING EXERCISE I

1. o
2. p
3. d
4. e
5. r
6. g
7. h
8. j
9. b
10. l
11. f
12. a
13. q
14. k
15. c
16. i
17. n
18. m

MATCHING EXERCISE II

1. r
2. m
3. n
4. j
5. a
6. q
7. d
8. c
9. f
10. k or p
11. b
12. g
13. o
14. e
15. l
16. h
17. p or k
18. i

▲ TEST YOUR KNOWLEDGE

1. pathogens
2. reservoir
3. virus
4. Airborne
5. immune system
6. asepsis
7. infectious
8. Diabetes
9. myocardial infarction
10. quadriplegia

Chapter 12

▲ KNOW YOUR TERMS

1. f
2. d
3. e
4. b
5. c
6. a
7. g

▲ TEST YOUR KNOWLEDGE

1. prefixes
2. roots
3. jargon
4. against
5. larynx
6. end
7. -algia
8. do not resuscitate
9. children
10. greater than

Chapter 13

▲ KNOW YOUR TERMS

1. m
2. o or h
3. n
4. b
5. l
6. c
7. a
8. p
9. k
10. d
11. g
12. j
13. h or o
14. e
15. f
16. i

▲ TEST YOUR KNOWLEDGE

1. objective
2. subjective
3. sender, receiver
4. end-of-shift
5. charting
6. nursing care plan
7. legal
8. flow sheet
9. graphic chart
10. Kardex

Chapter 14

▲ Know Your Terms

1. e
2. g
3. a
4. b
5. c
6. d
7. f

▲ Test Your Knowledge

1. raised
2. well lit
3. personal belongings
4. before, clean
5. after, dirty
6. closed
7. open or unoccupied
8. occupied
9. surgical
10. toe tuck

Chapter 15

▲ Know Your Terms

1. d
2. c
3. a
4. b

▲ Test Your Knowledge

1. Admission
2. admission chart
3. call signal
4. transfer
5. transfer
6. medical
7. discharge
8. ongoing
9. dietitian
10. referral

Chapter 16

KNOW YOUR TERMS

MATCHING EXERCISE I

1. d
2. g
3. m
4. h
5. f
6. a
7. j
8. n
9. b
10. c
11. i
12. k
13. e
14. l

MATCHING EXERCISE II

1. g
2. b
3. f
4. l
5. h
6. d
7. c
8. j
9. n
10. k
11. m
12. a
13. e
14. i

TEST YOUR KNOWLEDGE

1. Body mechanics
2. Body alignment
3. 12
4. friction
5. Draping
6. horizontal recumbent
7. transfer belt
8. mechanical lift
9. Range-of-motion
10. Abduction

Chapter 17

KNOW YOUR TERMS

1. f
2. d
3. g
4. b
5. c
6. e
7. a
8. i
9. k
10. h
11. j

TEST YOUR KNOWLEDGE

1. rehabilitation
2. breakdown
3. repetition
4. fractures
5. externally, internally
6. problems
7. infection
8. circulation
9. carry
10. prevent

CHAPTER 18

KNOW YOUR TERMS

1. f
2. h
3. a
4. b
5. d
6. c
7. i
8. e
9. g

TEST YOUR KNOWLEDGE

1. Hygiene
2. Oral hygiene
3. toothctte
4. Flossing
5. 105, 110
6. whirlpool
7. front, back
8. front, back
9. pressure sore or decubitus ulcer
10. sound

CHAPTER 19

KNOW YOUR TERMS

1. b
2. c
3. a

TEST YOUR KNOWLEDGE

1. atrophy
2. Elderly, geriatric
3. decreasing
4. drier
5. decrease
6. high-fiber
7. Reality orientation
8. confront
9. Dementia
10. Paranoid

CHAPTER 20

▲ KNOW YOUR TERMS

1. f
2. g
3. n
4. k
5. a
6. b
7. d
8. p
9. c
10. q
11. l
12. o
13. j
14. m
15. h
16. e
17. i

▲ TEST YOUR KNOWLEDGE

1. oral
2. tympanic
3. blood pressure
4. higher
5. radial
6. stethoscope
7. respiration
8. sphygmomanometer
9. Systolic
10. Diastolic

CHAPTER 21

▲ KNOW YOUR TERMS

1. m
2. f
3. n
4. a
5. c
6. j
7. k
8. d
9. b
10. l
11. g
12. e
13. h
14. i

▲ TEST YOUR KNOWLEDGE

1. Nutrition
2. protein
3. carbohydrates
4. six
5. Dehydration
6. NPO
7. graduate
8. Intravenous
9. Appetite
10. Anorexia

CHAPTER 22

KNOW YOUR TERMS

MATCHING EXERCISE I

1. n
2. l
3. a
4. s
5. q
6. m
7. e
8. d
9. b
10. h
11. f
12. i
13. g
14. k
15. j
16. c
17. o
18. r
19. p

MATCHING EXERCISE II

1. c
2. i
3. g
4. a
5. f
6. e
7. j
8. q
9. r
10. m
11. b
12. n
13. k
14. o
15. d
16. l
17. h
18. p

TEST YOUR KNOWLEDGE

1. Elimination
2. feces
3. Incontinence
4. constipation
5. flatulence
6. bedpan
7. catheter
8. clean-catch
9. glucose, ketones
10. enema

Chapter 23

▲ Know Your Terms

1. s
2. t
3. f
4. a
5. l
6. o
7. b
8. r
9. d
10. q
11. c
12. m
13. p
14. e
15. g
16. j
17. h
18. k
19. i
20. n

▲ Test Your Knowledge

1. carbohydrates
2. Hypoglycemia
3. Hyperglycemia
4. kidney dialysis
5. carcinoma
6. carcinogen
7. AIDS
8. cerebrovascular accident
9. Congestive heart failure
10. Parkinson's disease

Chapter 24

▲ Know Your Terms

1. c or h
2. e
3. a
4. b
5. c, d, or h
6. c, d, or h
7. f
8. g

▲ Test Your Knowledge

1. preoperative
2. consent
3. General
4. Local
5. Postoperative
6. 15
7. pneumonia
8. Atelectasis
9. thrombus
10. embolus

Chapter 25

▲ KNOW YOUR TERMS

1. f
2. a
3. h
4. b
5. d
6. c
7. e
8. g

▲ TEST YOUR KNOWLEDGE

1. compress
2. pack
3. aquamatic pad
4. decreases
5. increases
6. Sponge baths
7. immobilize
8. cyanosis
9. sitz bath
10. gauze

Chapter 26

▲ KNOW YOUR TERMS

1. c
2. d
3. b
4. a

▲ TEST YOUR KNOWLEDGE

1. housekeeping
2. independence
3. report
4. 911
5. clear
6. vacuuming
7. food preparation
8. nutrition
9. independence
10. Abandonment

CHAPTER 27

KNOW YOUR TERMS

1. l
2. m
3. k
4. c
5. n
6. h
7. j
8. g
9. d
10. a
11. e
12. b
13. i
14. f

TEST YOUR KNOWLEDGE

1. Maturity
2. Alzheimer's
3. sundowning
4. 3
5. psychosis
6. schizophrenia
7. abstinence
8. Anxiety
9. Agitation
10. Hallucinations

CHAPTER 28

KNOW YOUR TERMS

1. d
2. e
3. c or k
4. a
5. b
6. j
7. c or k
8. f
9. h
10. g
11. i

TEST YOUR KNOWLEDGE

1. Bonding
2. fontanels
3. 101° F
4. swaddled
5. colostrum
6. rooting
7. umbilical cord
8. Circumcision
9. burp
10. backs

Chapter 29

▲ KNOW YOUR TERMS

1. c
2. a
3. b

▲ TEST YOUR KNOWLEDGE

1. episiotomy
2. postpartum depression
3. areola
4. 10
5. letdown reflex
6. 500
7. Engorged
8. expressing
9. burp
10. overstimulate, irritate

Chapter 30

▲ KNOW YOUR TERMS

Any illness for which there is no cure and that eventually progresses to death.

▲ TEST YOUR KNOWLEDGE

1. terminal
2. Hospices
3. semi-Fowler's
4. bladder, bowel
5. decreased
6. mucus
7. psychological
8. false
9. gentle
10. AIDS

CHAPTER 31

▲ KNOW YOUR TERMS

1. g
2. e
3. f
4. b
5. c
6. d
7. h
8. a

▲ TEST YOUR KNOWLEDGE

1. Denial
2. Anger
3. Bargaining
4. Depression
5. Acceptance
6. Cheyne-Stokes
7. do not resuscitate
8. death
9. Rigor mortis
10. Postmortem